NERVES AND COMMON SENSE

BY

ANNIE PAYSON CALL

MANY of these articles first appeared in "The Ladies' Home Journal," and I am glad to take this opportunity of thanking Mr. Edward Bok—the editor—for his very helpful and suggestive titles.

ANNIE PAYSON CALL.

CONTENTS

I.	HABIT AND NERVOUS STRAIN	1
II.	HOW WOMEN CAN KEEP FROM BEING NERVOUS	3
III.	"YOU HAVE NO IDEA HOW I AM RUSHED"	14
IV.	"WHY DOES MRS. SMITH GET ON MY NERVES?"	23
V.	THE TRYING MEMBER OF THE FAMILY	32
VI.	IRRITABLE HUSBANDS	41
VII.	QUIET vs. CHRONIC EXCITEMENT	50
VIII.	THE TIRED EMPHASIS	58
IX.	HOW TO BE ILL AND GET WELL	63
X.	IS PHYSICAL CULTURE GOOD FOR GIRLS?	68
XI.	WORKING RESTFULLY	77
XII.	IMAGINARY VACATIONS	85
XIII.	THE WOMAN AT THE NEXT DESK	90
XIV.	TELEPHONES AND TELEPHONING	95
XV.	DON'T TALK	99
XVI.	"WHY FUSS SO MUCH ABOUT WHAT I EAT?"	104

XVII.	TAKE CARE OF YOUR STOMACH	113
XVIII.	ABOUT FACES	118
XIX.	ABOUT VOICES	121
XX.	ABOUT FRIGHTS	126
XXI.	CONTRARINESS	129
XXII.	HOW TO SEW EASILY	135
XXIII.	DO NOT HURRY	139
XXIV.	THE CARE OF AN INVALID	144
XXV.	THE HABIT OF ILLNESS	149
XXVI.	WHAT IS IT THAT MAKES ME SO NERVOUS?	157
XXVII.	POSITIVE AND NEGATIVE EFFORT	168
XXVIII.	HUMAN DUST	178
XXIX.	PLAIN EVERY-DAY COMMON SENSE	188
XXX.	A SUMMING UP	198

CHAPTER I

Habit and Nervous Strain

PEOPLE form habits which cause nervous strain. When these habits have fixed themselves for long enough upon their victims, the nerves give way and severe depression or some other form of nervous prostration is the result. If such an illness turns the attention to its cause, and so starts the sufferer toward a radical change from habits which cause nervous strain to habits which bring nervous strength, then the illness can be the beginning of better and permanent health. If, however, there simply is an enforced rest, without any intelligent understanding of the trouble, the invalid gets "well" only to drag out a miserable existence or to get very ill again.

Although any nervous suffering is worth while if it is the means of teaching us how to avoid nervous strain, it certainly is far preferable to avoid the strain without the extreme pain of a nervous breakdown.

To point out many of these pernicious habits and to suggest a practical remedy for each and all of them is the aim of this book, and for that reason common examples in various phases of every-day life are used as illustrations.

When there is no organic trouble there can be no doubt that *defects of character, inherited or acquired, are at the root of all nervous illness.* If this can once be generally recognized and acknowledged, especially by the sufferers themselves, we are in a fair way toward eliminating such illness entirely.

The trouble is people suffer from mortification and an unwillingness to look their bad habits in the face. They have not learned that humiliation can be wholesome, sound, and healthy, and so they keep themselves in a mess of a fog because they will not face the shame necessary to get out of it. They would rather be ill and suffering, and believe themselves to have strong characters than to look the weakness of their characters in the face, own up to them like men, and come out into open fresh air with healthy nerves which will gain in strength as they live.

Any intelligent man or woman who thinks a bit for himself can see the stupidity of this mistaken choice at a glance, and seeing it will act against it and thus do so much toward bringing light to all nervously prostrated humanity.

We can talk about faith cure, Christian Science, mind cure, hypnotism, psychotherapeutics, or any other forms of nerve cure which at the very best can only give the man a gentle shunt toward the middle of the stream of life. Once assured of the truth, the man must hold himself in the clean wholesomeness of it by actively working for his own strength of character *from his own initiative*. There can be no other permanent cure.

I say that strength of character must grow from our own initiative, and I should add that it must be from our own initiative that we come to recognize and actively believe that we are dependent upon a power not our own and our real strength comes from ceasing to be an obstruction to that power. The work of not interfering with our best health, moral and physical, means hard fighting and steady, never-ending vigilance. But it pays—it more than pays! And, it seems to me, this prevailing trouble of nervous strain which is so much with us now can be the means of guiding all men and women toward more solid health than has ever been known before. *But we must work for it!* We must give up expecting to be cured.

CHAPTER II

How Women can keep from being Nervous

MANY people suffer unnecessarily from "nerves" just for the want of a little knowledge of how to adjust themselves in order that the nerves may get well. As an example, I have in mind a little woman who had been ill for eight years—eight of what might have been the best years of her life—all because neither she nor her family knew the straight road toward getting well. Now that she has found the path she has gained health wonderfully in six months, and promises to be better than ever before in her life.

Let me tell you how she became ill and then I can explain her process of getting well again. One night she was overtired and could not get to sleep, and became very much annoyed at various noises that were about the house. Just after she had succeeded in stopping one noise she would go back to bed and hear several others. Finally, she was so worked up and nervously strained over the noises that her hearing became exaggerated, and she was troubled by noises that other people would not have even heard; so she managed to keep herself awake all night.

The next day the strain of the overfatigue was, of course, very much increased, not only by the wakeful night, but also by the annoyance which had kept her awake. The family were distressed that she should not have slept all night; talked a great deal about it, and called in the doctor.

The woman's strained nerves were on edge all day, so that her feelings were easily hurt, and her brothers and sisters became, as they thought, justly impatient at what they considered her silly babyishness. This, of course, roused her to more strain. The overcare and the feeble, unintelligent sympathy that she had from some members of her family kept her weak and self-centered, and the ignorant, selfish impatience with which the others treated her increased her nervous strain. After this there followed various other worries and a personal sense of annoyance—all of which made her more nervous.

Then—the stomach and brain are so closely associated—her digestion began to cause her discomfort: a lump in her stomach, her food "would not digest," and various other symptoms, all of which mean strained and overwrought nerves, although they are more often attributed merely to a disordered stomach. She worried as to what she had better eat and what she had better not eat. If her stomach was tired and some simple food disagreed with her all the discomfort was attributed to the food, instead of to the real cause,—a tired stomach,—and the cause back of that,—strained nerves. The consequence was that one kind of wholesome food after another was cut off as being impossible for her to eat. Anything that this poor little invalid did not like about circumstances or people she felt ugly and cried over. Finally, the entire family were centered about her illness, either in overcare or annoyance.

You see, she kept constantly repeating her brain impression of overfatigue: first annoyance because she stayed awake; then annoyance at noises; then excited distress that she should have stayed awake all night; then resistance and anger at other people who interfered with her. Over and over that brain impression of nervous illness was repeated by the woman herself and people about her until she seemed settled into it for the rest of her life. It was like expecting a sore to get well while it was constantly being rubbed and irritated. A woman might have the healthiest blood in the world, but if she cut herself and then rubbed and irritated the cut, and put salt in it, it would be impossible for it to heal.

Now let me tell you how this little woman got well. The first thing she did was to take some very simple relaxing exercises while she was lying in bed. She raised her arms very slowly and as loosely as she could from the elbow and then her hands from the wrist, and stretched and relaxed her fingers steadily, then dropped her hand and forearm heavily, and felt it drop slowly at first, then quickly and quietly, with its own weight. She tried to shut her eyes like a baby going to sleep, and followed that with long, gentle, quiet breaths. These and other exercises gave her an impression of quiet relaxation so that she became more sensitive to superfluous tension.

When she felt annoyed at noises she easily noticed that in response to the annoyance her whole body became tense and strained. After she had done her exercises and felt quiet and rested something would happen or some one would say something that went against the grain, and quick as a wink all the good of the exercises would be gone and she would be tight and strained again, and nervously irritated.

Very soon she saw clearly that she must learn to drop the habit of physical strain if she wanted to get well; but she also learned what was more—far more—important than that: that *she must conquer the cause of the strain or she could never permanently drop it.* She saw that the cause was resentment and resistance to the noises—the circumstances, the people, and all the variety of things that had "made her nervous."

Then she began her steady journey toward strong nerves and a wholesome, happy life. She began the process of changing her brain impressions. If she heard noises that annoyed her she would use her will to direct her attention toward dropping resistance to the noises, and in order to drop her mental resistance she gave her attention to loosening out the bodily contractions. Finally she became interested in the new process as in a series of deep and true experiments. Of course her living and intelligent interest enabled her to gain very much faster, for she not only enjoyed her growing freedom, but she also enjoyed seeing her experiments work. Nature always tends toward health, and if we stop interfering with her she will get us well.

There is just this difference between the healing of a physical sore and the healing of strained and irritated nerves

With the one our bodies are healed, and things go on in them about the same as before. With the other, every use of the will to free ourselves from the irritation and its cause not only enables us to get free from the nervous illness, but in addition brings us new nerve vigor.

When nervous illness is met deeply enough and in the normal way, the result is that the nerves become stronger than ever before.

Often the effect of nervous strain in women is constant talking. Talk—talk—talk, and mostly about themselves, their ailments, their worries, and the hindrances that are put in their way to prevent their getting well. This talking is not a relief, as people sometimes feel. It is a direct waste of vigor. But the waste would be greater if the talk were repressed. The only real help comes when the talker herself recognizes the strain of her talk and "loosens" into silence.

People must find themselves out to get well—really well—from nervous suffering. The cause of nervous strain is so often in the character and in the way we meet circumstances and people that it seems essential to recognize our mistakes in that direction, and to face them squarely before we can do our part toward removing the causes of any nervous illness.

Remember it is not circumstances that keep us ill. It is not people that cause our illness. It is not our environment that overcomes us. It is the way we face and deal with circumstances, with people, and with environment that keeps our nerves irritated or keeps them quiet and wholesome and steady.

Let me tell the story of two men, both of whom were brought low by severe nervous breakdown. One complained of his environment, complained of circumstances, complained of people. Everything and every one was the cause of his suffering, except himself. The result was that he weakened his brain by the constant willful and enforced strain, so that what little health he regained was the result of Nature's steady and powerful tendency toward health, and in spite of the man himself.

The other man—to give a practical instance—returned from a journey taken in order to regain the strength which he had lost from not knowing how to work. His business agent met him at the railroad station with a piece of very bad news. Instead of being frightened and resisting and contracting in every nerve of his body, he took it at once as an opportunity to drop resistance. He had learned to relax his body, and by doing relaxing and quieting exercises over and over he had given himself a brain impression of quiet and "let go" which he could recall at will. Instead of expressing distress at the bad news he used his will at once to drop resistance and relax; and, to the surprise of his informant, who had felt that he must break his bad news as easily as possible, he said "Anything else?" Yes, there was another piece of news about as bad as the first. "Go on," answered the man who had been sick with nerves; "tell me something else."

And so he did, until he had told him five different things which were about as disagreeable and painful to hear as could have been. For every bit of news our friend used his will with decision to drop the resistance, which would, of course, at once arise in response to all that seemed to go against him.

He had, of course, to work at intervals for long afterward to keep free from the resistance; but the habit is getting more and more established as life goes on with him, and the result is a brain clearer than ever before in his life, a power of nerve which is a surprise to every one about him, and a most successful business career.

The success in business is, however, a minor matter. His brain would have cleared and his nerve strengthened just the same if what might be called the business luck had continued to go against him, as it seemed to do for the first few months after his recovery. That everything did go against him for some time was the greatest blessing he could have had. The way he met all the reverses increased his nerve power steadily and consistently.

These two men are fair examples of two extremes. The first one did not know how to meet life. If he had had the opportunity to learn he might have done as well as the other. The second had worked and studied to help himself out of nerves, and had found the true secret of doing it.

Some men, however, and, I regret to say, more women, have the weakening habit so strong upon them that they are unwilling to learn how to get well, even when they have the opportunity. It seems so strange to see people suffer intensely—and be unwilling to face and follow the only way that will lead them out of their torture.

The trouble is we want our own way and nervous health, too, and with those who have once broken down nervously the only chance of permanent health is through learning to drop the strain of resistance when things do not go their way. This is proved over and over by the constant relapse into "nerves" which comes to those who have simply been healed over. Even with those who appear to have been well for some time, if they have not acquired the habit of dropping their mental and physical tension you can always detect an overcare for themselves which means dormant fear—or even active fear in the background.

There are some wounds which the surgeons keep open, even though the process is most painful, because they know that to heal really they must heal from the inside. Healing over on the outside only means decay underneath, and eventual death. This is in most cases exactly synonymous with the healing of broken-down nerves. They must be healed in causes to be permanently cured. Sometimes the change that comes in the process is so great that it is like reversing an engine.

If the little woman whom I mentioned first had practiced relaxing and quieting exercises every day for years, and had not used the quiet impression gained by the exercises to help her in dropping mental resistances, she never would have gained her health.

Concentrating steadily on dropping the tension of the body is very radically helpful in dropping resistance from the mind, and the right idea is to do the exercises over and over until the impression of quiet openness is, by constant repetition, so strong with us that we can recall it at will whenever we need it. Finally, after repeated tests, we gain the habit of meeting the difficulties of life without strain—first in little ways, and then in larger ways.

The most quieting, relaxing, and strengthening of all exercises for the nerves comes in deep and rhythmic breathing, and in voice exercises in connection with it. Nervous strain is more evident in a voice than in any other expressive part of man or woman. It sometimes seems as if all other relaxing exercises were mainly useful because of opening a way for us to breathe better. There is a pressure on every part of the body when we inhale, and a consequent reaction when we exhale, and the more passive the body is when we take our deep breaths the more freely and quietly the blood can circulate all the way through it, and, of course, all nervous and muscular contraction impairs circulation, and all impaired circulation emphasizes nervous contraction.

To any one who is suffering from "nerves," in a lesser or greater degree, it could not fail to be of very great help to take half an hour in the morning, lie flat on the back, with the body as loose and heavy as it can be made, and then study taking gentle, quiet, and rhythmic breaths, long and short. Try to have the body so loose and open and responsive that it will open as you inhale and relax as you exhale, just as a rubber bag would. Of course, it will take time, but the refreshing quiet is sure to come if the practice is repeated regularly for a long enough time, and eventually we would no more miss it than we would go without our dinner.

We must be careful after each deep, long breath to rest quietly and let our lungs do as they please. Be careful to begin the breaths delicately and gently, to inhale with the same gentleness with which we begin, and to make the change from inhaling to exhaling with the greatest delicacy possible—keeping the body loose.

For the shorter breaths we can count three, or five, or ten to inhale, and the same number to exhale, until we have the rhythm established, and then go on breathing without counting, as if we were sound asleep. Always aim for gentleness and delicacy. If we have not half an hour to spare to lie quietly and breathe we can practice the breathing while we walk. It is wonderful how we detect strain and resistance in our breath, and the restfulness which comes when we breathe so gently that the breath seems to come and go without our volition brings new life with it.

We must expect to gain slowly and be patient; we must remember that nerves always get well by ups and downs, and use our wills to make every down lead to a higher up. If we want the lasting benefit, or any real benefit at all when we get the brain impression of quiet freedom from these breathing exercises, we must insist upon recalling that impression every time a test comes, and face the circumstances, or the person, or the duty with a voluntary insistence upon a quiet, open brain, rather than a tense, resistant one.

It will come hard at first, but we are sure to get there if we keep steadily at it, for it is really the Law of the Lord God Almighty that we are learning to obey, and this process of learning gives us steadily an enlarged appreciation of what trust in the Lord really is. There is no trust without obedience, and an intelligent obedience begets trust. The nerves touch the soul on one side and the body on the other, and we must work for freedom of soul and body in response to spiritual and physical law if we want to get sick nerves well. If we do not remember always a childlike attitude toward the Lord the best nerve training is only an easy way of being selfish.

To sum it all up—if you want to learn to help yourself out of "nerves" learn to rest when you rest and to work without strain when you work; learn to loosen out of the muscular contractions which the nerves cause; learn to drop the mental resistances which cause the "nerves," and which take the form of anger, resentment, worry, anxiety, impatience, annoyance, or self-pity; eat only nourishing food, eat it slowly, and chew it well; breathe the freshest air you can, and breathe it deeply, gently, and rhythmically; take what healthy, vigorous exercise you find possible; do your daily work to the best of your ability; give your attention so entirely to the process of gaining health for the sake of your work and other people that you have no mind left with which to complain of being ill, and see that all this effort aims toward a more intelligent obedience to and trustfulness in the Power that gives us life. Wholesome, sustained concentration is in the very essence of healthy nerves.

CHAPTER III

"You Have no Idea how I am Rushed"

A WOMAN can feel rushed when she is sitting perfectly still and has really nothing whatever to do. A woman can feel at leisure when she is working diligently at something, with a hundred other things waiting to be done when the time comes. It is not all we have to do that gives us the rushed feeling; it is the way we do what is before us. It is the attitude we take toward our work.

Now this rushed feeling in the brain and nerves is intensely oppressive. Many women, and men too, suffer from it keenly, and they suffer the more because they do not recognize that that feeling of rush is really entirely distinct from what they have to do; in truth it has nothing whatever to do with it.

I have seen a woman suffer painfully with the sense of being pushed for time when she had only two things to do in the whole day, and those two things at most need not take more than an hour each. This same woman was always crying for rest. I never knew, before I saw her, that women could get just as abnormal in their efforts to rest as in their insistence upon overwork. This little lady never rested when she went to rest; she would lie on the bed for hours in a state of strain about resting that was enough to tire any ordinarily healthy woman. One friend used to tell her that she was an inebriate on resting. It is perhaps needless to say that she was a nervous invalid, and in the process of gaining her health she had to be set to work and kept at work. Many and many a time she has cried and begged for rest when it was not rest she needed at all: it was work.

She has started off to some good, healthy work crying and sobbing at the cruelty that made her go, and has returned from the work as happy and healthy, apparently, as a little child. Then she could go to rest and rest to some purpose. She had been busy in wholesome action and the normal reaction came in her rest. As she grew more naturally interested in her work she rested less and less, and she rested better and better because she had something to rest from and something to rest for.

Now she does only a normal amount of resting, but gets new life from every moment of rest she takes; before, all her rest only made her want more rest and kept her always in the strain of fatigue. And what might seem to many a very curious result is that as the abnormal desire for rest disappeared the rushed feeling disappeared, too.

There is no one thing that American women need more than a healthy habit of rest, but it has got to be real rest, not strained nor self-indulgent rest.

Another example of this effort at rest which is a sham and a strain is the woman who insists upon taking a certain time every day in which to rest. She insists upon doing everything quietly and with—as she thinks—a sense of leisure, and yet she keeps the whole household in a sense of turmoil and does not know it. She sits complacently in her pose of prompt action, quietness and rest, and has a tornado all about her. She is so deluded in her own idea of herself that she does not observe the tornado, and yet she has caused it. Everybody in her household is tired out with her demands, and she herself is ill, chronically ill. But she thinks she is at peace, and she is annoyed that others should be tired.

If this woman could open and let out her own interior tornado, which she has kept frozen in there by her false attitude of restful quiet, she would be more ill for a time, but it might open her eyes to the true state of things and enable her to rest to some purpose and to allow her household to rest, too.

It seems, at first thought, strange that in this country, when the right habit of rest is so greatly needed, that the strain of rest should have become in late years one of the greatest defects. On second thought, however, we see that it is a perfectly rational result. We have strained to work and strained to play and strained to live for so long that when the need for rest gets so imperative that we feel we must rest the habit of strain is so upon us that we strain to rest. And what does such "rest" amount to? What strength does it bring us? What enlightenment do we get from it?

With the little lady of whom I first spoke rest was a steadily-weakening process. She was resting her body straight toward its grave. When a body rests and rests the circulation gets more and more sluggish until it breeds disease in the weakest organ, and then the physicians seem inclined to give their attention to the disease, and not to the cause of the abnormal strain which was behind the disease. Again, as we have seen, the abnormal, rushed feeling can exist just as painfully with too much and the wrong kind of rest as with too much work and the wrong way of working.

We have been, as a nation, inclined toward "Americanitis" for so long now that children and children's children have inherited a sense of rush, and they suffer intensely from it with a perfectly clear understanding of the fact that they have nothing whatever to hurry about. This is quite as true of men as it is of women. In such cases the first care should be not to fasten this sense of rush on to anything; the second care should be to go to work to cure it, to relax out of that contraction—just as you would work to cure twitching St. Vitus's dance, or any other nervous habit.

Many women will get up and dress in the morning as if they had to catch a train, and they will come in to breakfast as if it were a steamer for the other side of the world that they had to get, and no other steamer went for six months. They do not know that they are in a rush and a hurry, and they do not find it out until the strain has been on them for so long that they get nervously ill from it—and then they find themselves suffering from "that rushed feeling."

Watch some women in an argument pushing, actually rushing, to prove themselves right; they will hardly let their opponent have an opportunity to speak, much less will they stop to consider what he says and see if by chance he may not be right and they wrong.

The rushing habit is not by any means in the fact of doing many things. It asserts itself in our brains in talking, in writing, in thinking. How many of us, I wonder, have what might be called a quiet working brain? Most of us do not even know the standard of a brain that thinks and talks and lives quietly: a brain that never pushes and never rushes, or, if by any chance it is led into pushing or rushing, is so wholesomely sensitive that it drops the push or the rush as a bare hand would drop a red-hot coal.

None of us can appreciate the weakening power of this strained habit of rush until we have, by the use of our own wills, directed our minds toward finding a normal habit of quiet, and yet I do not in the least exaggerate when I say that its weakening effect on the brain and nerves is frightful.

And again I repeat, the rushed feeling has nothing whatever to do with the work before us. A woman can feel quite as rushed when she has nothing to do as when she is extremely busy.

"But," some one says, "may I not feel pressed for time when I have more to do than I can possibly put into the time before me?"

Oh, yes, yes—you can feel normally pressed for time; and because of this pressure you can arrange in your mind what best to leave undone, and so relieve the pressure. If one thing seems as important to do as another you can make up your mind that of course you can only do what you have time for, and the remainder must go. You cannot do what you have time to do so well if you are worrying about what you have no time for. There need be no abnormal sense of rush about it.

Just as Nature tends toward health, Nature tends toward rest—toward the right kind of rest; and if we have lost the true knack of resting we can just as surely find it as a sunflower can find the sun. It is not something artificial that we are trying to learn—it is something natural and alive, something that belongs to us, and our own best instinct will come to our aid in finding it if we will only first turn our attention toward finding our own best instinct.

We must have something to rest from, and we must have something to rest for, if we want to find the real power of rest. Then we must learn to let go of our nerves and our muscles, to leave everything in our bodies open and passive so that our circulation can have its own best way. But we must have had some activity in order to have given our circulation a fair start before we can expect it to do its best when we are passive.

Then, what is most important, we must learn to drop all effort of our minds if we want to know how to rest; and that is difficult. We can do it best by keeping our minds concentrated on something simple and quiet and wholesome. For instance, you feel tired and rushed and you can have half an hour in which to rest and get rid of the rush. Suppose you lie down on the bed and imagine yourself a turbulent lake after a storm. The storm is dying down, dying down, until by and by there is no wind, only little dashing waves that the wind has left. Then the waves quiet down steadily, more and more, until finally they are only ripples on the water. Then no ripples, but the water is as still as glass. The sun goes down. The sky glows. Twilight comes. One star appears, and green banks and trees and sky and stars are all reflected in the quiet mirror of the lake, and you are the lake, and you are quiet and refreshed and rested and ready to get up and go on with your work—to go on with it, too, better and more quietly than when you left it.

Or, another way to quiet your mind and to let your imagination help you to a better rest is to float on the top of a turbulent sea and then to sink down, down, down until you get into the still water at the bottom of the sea. We all know that, no matter how furious the sea is on the surface, not far below the surface it is absolutely still. It is very restful to go down there in imagination.

Whatever choice we may make to quiet our minds and our bodies, as soon as we begin to concentrate we must not be surprised if intruding thoughts are at first constantly crowding to get in. We must simply let them come. Let them come, and pay no attention to them.

I knew of a woman who was nervously ill, and some organs of her body were weakened very much by the illness. She made-up her mind to rest herself well and she did so. Every day she would rest for three hours; she said to herself, "I will rest an hour on my left side, an hour on my right side, and an hour on my back." And she did that for days and days. When she lay on one side she had a very attractive tree to look at. When she lay on the other she had an interesting picture before her. When she lay on her back she had the sky and several trees to see through a window in front of the bed. She grew steadily better every week—she had something to rest for. She was resting to get well. If she had rested and complained of her illness I doubt if she would have been well to-day. She simply refused to take the unpleasant sensations into consideration except for the sake of resting out of them. When she was well enough to take a little active exercise she knew she could rest better and get well faster for that, and she insisted upon taking the exercise, although at first she had to do it with the greatest care. Now that this woman is well she knows how to rest and she knows how to work better than ever before.

For normal rest we need the long sleep of night. For shorter rests which we may take during the day, often opportunity comes at most unexpected times and in most unexpected ways, and we must be ready to take advantage of it. We need also the habit of working restfully. This habit of course enables us to rest truly when we are only resting, and again the habit of resting normally helps us to work normally.

A wise old lady said: "My dear, you cannot exaggerate the unimportance of things." She expressed even more, perhaps, than she knew.

It is our habit of exaggerating the importance of things that keeps us hurried and rushed. It is our habit of exaggerating the importance of ourselves that makes us hold the strain of life so intensely. If we would be content to do one thing at a time, and concentrate on that one thing until it came time to do the next thing, it would astonish us to see how much we should accomplish. A healthy concentration is at the root of working restfully and of resting restfully, for a healthy concentration means dropping everything that interferes.

I know there are women who read this article who will say; "Oh, yes, that is all very well for some women, but it does not apply in the least to a woman who has my responsibilities, or to a woman who has to work as I have to work."

My answer to that is: "Dear lady, you are the very one to whom it does apply!"

The more work we have to do, the harder our lives are, the more we need the best possible principles to lighten our work and to enlighten our lives. We are here in the world at school and we do not want to stay in the primary classes.

The harder our lives are and the more we are handicapped the more truly we can learn to make every limitation an opportunity—and if we persistently do that through circumstances, no matter how severe, the nearer we are to getting our diploma. To gain our freedom from the rushed feeling, to find a quiet mind in place of an unquiet one, is worth working hard for through any number of difficulties. And think of the benefit such a quiet mind could be to other people! Especially if the quiet mind were the mind of a woman, for, at the present day, think what a contrast she would be to other women!

When a woman's mind is turbulent it is the worst kind of turbulence. When it is quiet we can almost say it is the best kind of quiet, humanly speaking.

CHAPTER IV

Why does Mrs. Smith get on My Nerves?

IF you want to know the true answer to this question it is "because you are unwilling that Mrs. Smith should be herself." You want her to be just like you, or, if not just like you, you want her to be just as you would best like her.

I have seen a woman so annoyed that she could not eat her supper because another woman ate sugar on baked beans. When this woman told me later what it was that had taken away her appetite she added: "And isn't it absurd? Why shouldn't Mrs. Smith eat sugar on baked beans? It does not hurt me. I do not have to taste the sugar on the beans; but is it such an odd thing to do. It seems to me such bad manners that I just get so mad I can't eat!"

Now, could there be anything more absurd than that? To see a woman annoyed; to see her recognize that she was uselessly and foolishly annoyed, and yet to see that she makes not the slightest effort to get over her annoyance.

It is like the woman who discovered that she spoke aloud in church, and was so surprised that she exclaimed: "Why, I spoke out loud in church!" and then, again surprised, she cried: "Why, I keep speaking aloud in church!"—and it did not occur to her to stop.

My friend would have refused an invitation to supper, I truly believe, if she had known that Mrs. Smith would be there and her hostess would have baked beans. She was really a slave to Mrs. Smith's way of eating baked beans.

"Well, I do not blame her," I hear some reader say; "it is entirely out of place to eat sugar on baked beans. Why shouldn't she be annoyed?"

I answer: "Why should she be annoyed? Will her annoyance stop Mrs. Smith's eating sugar on baked beans? Will she in any way—selfish or otherwise—be the gainer for her annoyance? Furthermore, if it were the custom to eat sugar on baked beans, as it is the custom to put sugar in coffee, this woman would not have been annoyed at all. It was simply the fact of seeing Mrs. Smith digress from the ordinary course of life that annoyed her."

It is the same thing that makes a horse shy. The horse does not say to himself, "There is a large carriage, moving with no horse to pull it, with nothing to push it, with—so far as I can see—no motive power at all. How weird that is! How frightful!"—and, with a quickly beating heart, jump aside and caper in scared excitement. A horse when he first sees an automobile gets an impression on his brain which is entirely out of his ordinary course of impressions—it is as if some one suddenly and unexpectedly struck him, and he shies and jumps. The horse is annoyed, but he does not know what it is that annoys him. Now, when a horse shies you drive him away from the automobile and quiet him down, and then, if you are a good trainer, you drive him back again right in front of that car or some other one, and you repeat the process until the automobile becomes an ordinary impression to him, and he is no longer afraid of it.

There is, however, just this difference between a woman and a horse: the woman has her own free will behind her annoyance, and a horse has not. If my friend had asked Mrs. Smith to supper twice a week, and had served baked beans each time and herself passed her the sugar with careful courtesy, and if she had done it all deliberately for the sake of getting over her annoyance, she would probably have only increased it until the strain would have got on her nerves much more seriously than Mrs. Smith ever had. Not only that, but she would have found herself resisting other people's peculiarities more than ever before; I have seen people in nervous prostration from causes no more serious than that, on the surface. It is the habit of resistance and resentment back of the surface annoyance which is the serious cause of many a woman's attack of nerves.

Every woman is a slave to every other woman who annoys her. She is tied to each separate woman who has got on her nerves by a wire which is pulling, pulling the nervous force right out of her. And it is not the other woman's fault—it is her own. The wire is pulling, whether or not we are seeing or thinking of the other woman, for, having once been annoyed by her, the contraction is right there in our brains. It is just so much deposited strain in our nervous systems which will stay there until we, of our own free wills, have yielded out of it.

The horse was not resenting nor resisting the automobile; therefore the strain of his fright was at once removed when the automobile became an ordinary impression. A woman, when she gets a new impression that she does not like, resents and resists it with her will, and she has got to get in behind that resistance and drop it with her will before she is a free woman.

To be sure, there are many disagreeable things that annoy for a time, and then, as the expression goes, we get hardened to them. But few of us know that this hardening is just so much packed resistance which is going to show itself later in some unpleasant form and make us ill in mind or body. We have got to yield, yield, yield out of every bit of resistance and resentment to other people if we want to be free. No reasoning about it is going to do us any good. No passing back and forth in front of it is going to free us. We must yield first and then we can see clearly and reason justly. We must yield first and then we can go back and forth in front of it, and it will only be a reminder to yield every time until the habit of yielding has become habitual and the strength of nerve and strength of character developed by means of the yielding have been established.

Let me explain more fully what I mean by "yielding." Every annoyance, resistance, or feeling of resentment contracts us in some way physically; if we turn our attention toward dropping that physical contraction, with a real desire to get rid of the resistance behind it, we shall find that dropping the physical strain opens the way to drop the mental and moral strain, and when we have really dropped the strain we invariably find reason and justice and even generosity toward others waiting to come to us.

There is one important thing to be looked out for in this normal process of freeing ourselves from other people. A young girl said once to her teacher: "I got mad the other day and I relaxed, and the more I relaxed the madder I got!"

"Did you want to get over the anger?" asked the teacher.

"No, I didn't," was the prompt and ready answer.

Of course, as this child relaxed out of the tension of her anger, there was only more anger to take its place, and the more she relaxed the more free her nerves were to take the impression of the anger hoarded up in her; consequently it was as she said: the more she relaxed the "madder" she got. Later, this same little girl came to understand fully that she must have a real desire to get over her anger in order to have better feelings come up after she had dropped the contraction of the anger.

I know of a woman who has been holding such steady hatred for certain other people that the strain of it has kept her ill. And it is all a matter of feeling: first, that these people have interfered with her welfare; second, that they differ from her in opinion. Every once in a while her hatred finds a vent and spends itself in tears and bitter words. Then, after the external relief of letting out her pent-up feeling, she closes up again and one would think from her voice and manner—if one did not look very deep in—that she had only kindliness for every one. But she stays nervously ill right along.

How could she do otherwise with that strain in her? If she were constitutionally a strong woman this strain of hatred would have worn on her, though possibly not have made her really ill; but, being naturally sensitive and delicate, the strain has kept her an invalid altogether.

"Mother, I can't stand Maria," one daughter says to her mother, and when inquiry is made the mother finds that what her daughter "cannot stand" is ways that differ from her own. Sometimes, however, they are very disagreeable ways which are exactly like the ways of the person who cannot stand them. If one person is imperious and demanding she will get especially annoyed at another person for being imperious and demanding, without a suspicion that she is objecting vehemently to a reflection of herself.

There are two ways in which people get on our nerves. The first way lies in their difference from us in habit—in little things and in big things; their habits are not our habits. Their habits may be all right, and our habits may be all right, but they are "different." Why should we not be willing to have them different? Is there any reason for it except the very empty one that we consciously and unconsciously want every one else to be just like us, or to believe just as we do, or to behave just as we do? And what sense is there in that?

"I cannot stand Mrs. So-and-so; she gets into a rocking-chair and rocks and rocks until I feel as if I should go crazy!" some one says. But why not let Mrs. So-and-so rock? It is her chair while she is in it, and her rocking. Why need it touch us at all?

"But," I hear a hundred women say, "it gets on our nerves; how can we help its getting on our nerves?" The answer to that is: "Drop it off your nerves." I know many women who have tried it and who have succeeded, and who are now profiting by the relief. Sometimes the process to such freedom is a long one; sometimes it is a short one; but, either way, the very effort toward it brings nervous strength, as well as strength of character.

Take the woman who rocks. Practically every time she rocks you should relax, actually and consciously relax your muscles and your nerves. The woman who rocks need not know you are relaxing; it all can be done from inside. Watch and you will find your muscles strained and tense with resistance to the rocking. Go to work practically to drop every bit of strain that you observe. As you drop the grossest strain it will make you more sensitive to the finer strain and you can drop that—and it is even possible that you may seek the woman who rocks, in order to practice on her and get free from the habit of resisting more quickly.

This seems comical—almost ridiculous—to think of seeking an annoyance in order to get rid of it; but, after laughing at it first, look at the idea seriously, and you will see it is common sense. When you have learned to relax to the woman who rocks you have learned to relax to other similar annoyances. You have been working on a principle that applies generally. You have acquired a good habit which can never really fail you.

If my friend had invited Mrs. Smith to supper and served baked beans for the sake of relaxing out of the tension of her resistance to the sugar, then she could have conquered that resistance. But to try to conquer an annoyance like that without knowing how to yield in some way would be, so far as I know, an impossibility. Of course, we would prefer that our friends should not have any disagreeable, ill-bred, personal ways, but we can go through the world without resisting them, and there is no chance of helping any one out of them through our own resistances.

On the other hand a way may open by which the woman's attention is called to the very unhealthy habit of rocking—or eating sugar on beans—if we are ready, without resistance, to point it out to her. And if no way opens we have at least put ourselves out of bondage to her. The second way in which other people get on our nerves is more serious and more difficult. Mrs. So-and-so may be doing very wrong—really very wrong; or some one who is nearly related to us may be doing very wrong—and it may be our most earnest and sincere desire to set him right. In such cases the strain is more intense because we really have right on our side, in our opinion, if not in our attitude toward the other person. Then, to recognize that if some one else chooses to do wrong it is none of our business is one of the most difficult things to do—for a woman, especially.

It is more difficult to recognize practically that, in so far as it may be our business, we can best put ourselves in a position to enable the other person to see his own mistake by dropping all personal resistance to it and all personal strain about it. Even a mother with her son can help him to be a man much more truly if she stops worrying about and resisting his unmanliness.

"But," I hear some one say, "that all seems like such cold indifference." Not at all—not at all. Such freedom from strain can be found only through a more actively affectionate interest in others. The more we truly love another, the more thoroughly we respect that other's individuality.

The other so-called love is only love of possession and love of having our own way. It is not really love at all; it is sugar-coated tyranny. And when one sugar-coated tyrant' antagonizes herself against another sugar-coated tyrant the strain is severe indeed, and nothing good is ever accomplished.

The Roman infantry fought with a fixed amount of space about each soldier, and found that the greater freedom of individual activity enabled them to fight better and to conquer their foes. This symbolizes happily the process of getting people off our nerves. Let us give each one a wide margin and thus preserve a good margin for ourselves.

We rub up against other people's nerves by getting too near to them—not too near to their real selves, but too near, so to speak, to their nervous systems. There have been quarrels between good people just because one phase of nervous irritability roused another. Let things in other people go until you have entirely dropped your strain about them—then it will be clear enough what to do and what to say, or what not to do and what not to say. People in the world cannot get on our nerves unless we allow them to do so.

CHAPTER V

The Trying Member of the Family

"TOMMY, don't do that. You know it annoys your grandfather."

"Well, why should he be annoyed? I am doing nothing wrong."

"I know that, and it hurts me to ask you, but you know how he will feel if he sees you doing it, and you know that troubles me."

Reluctantly and sullenly Tommy stopped. Tommy's mother looked strained and worried and discontented. Tommy had an expression on his face akin to that of a smouldering volcano.

If any one had taken a good look at the grandfather it would have been very clear that Tommy was his own grandson, and that the old man and the child were acting and reacting upon one another in a way that was harmful to both; although the injury was, of course, worse to the child, for the grandfather had toughened. The grandfather thought he loved his little grandson, and the grandson, at times, would not have acknowledged that he did not love his grandfather. At other times, with childish frankness, he said he "hated him."

But the worst of this situation was that although the mother loved her son, and loved her father, and sincerely thought that she was the family peacemaker, she was all the time fanning the antagonism.

Here is a contrast to this little story An old uncle came into the family of his nephew to live, late in life, and with a record behind him of whims and crotchets in the extreme. The father and mother talked it over. Uncle James must come. He had lost all his money. There was no one else to look after him and they could not afford to support him elsewhere where he would be comfortable. They took it into account, without offence, that it was probably just as much a cross to Uncle James to come as it was to them to have him. They took no pose of magnanimity such as: "Of course we must be good and offer Uncle James a home," and "How good we are to do it!" Uncle James was to come because it was the only thing for him to do. The necessity was to be faced and fought and conquered, and they had three strong, self-willed little children to face it with them. They had sense enough to see that if faced rightly it would do only good to the children, but if made a burden to groan over it would make their home a "hornets' nest." They agreed to say nothing to the children about Uncle James's peculiarities, but to await developments.

Children are always delighted at a visit from a relative, and they welcomed their great-uncle with pleasure. It was not three days, however, before every one of the three was crying with dislike and hurt feelings and anger. Then was the time to begin the campaign.

The mother, with a happy face, called the three children to her, and said "Now listen, children. Do you suppose I like Uncle James's irritability any better than you do?"

"No," came in a chorus; "we don't see how you stand it, Mother."

Then she said: "Now look here, boys, do you suppose that Uncle James likes his snapping any better than we do?"

"If he does not like it why does he do it?" answered the boys.

"I cannot tell you that; that is his business and not yours or mine," said the mother; "but I can prove to you that he does not like it. Bobby, do you remember how you snapped at your brother yesterday, when he accidentally knocked your house over?"

"Yes!" replied Bobby.

"Did you feel comfortable after it?" "You bet I didn't," was the quick reply.

"Well," answered the mother, "you boys stop and think just how disagreeable it is inside of you when you snap, and then think how it would be if you had to feel like that as much as Uncle James does."

"By golly, but that would be bad," said the twelve-year-old.

"Now, boys," went on the mother, "you want to relieve Uncle James's disagreeable feelings all you can, and don't you see that you increase them when you do things to annoy him? His snappish feelings are just like a sore that is smarting and aching all the time, and when you get in their way it hurts as if you rubbed the sore. Keep out of his way when you can, and when you can't and he snaps at you, say: 'I beg your pardon, sir,' like gentlemen, and stop doing what annoys him; or get out of his way as soon as you can."

Uncle James never became less snappish. But the upright, manly courtesy of those boys toward him was like fresh air on a mountain, especially because it had become a habit and was all as a matter of course. The father and mother realized that Uncle James had, unconsciously, made men of their boys as nothing else in the world could have done, and had trained them so that they would grow up tolerant and courteous toward all human peculiarities.

Many times a gracious courtesy toward the "trying member" will discover good and helpful qualities that we had not guessed before. Sometimes after a little honest effort we find that it is ourselves who have been the trying members, and that the other one has been the member tried. Often it is from two members of the family that the trying element comes. Two sisters may clash, and they will generally clash because they are unlike. Suppose one sister moves and lives in big swings, and the other in minute details. Of course when these extreme tendencies are accented in each the selfish temptation is for the larger mind to lapse into carelessness of details, and for the smaller mind to shrink into pettiness, and as this process continues the sisters get more and more intolerant of each other, and farther and farther apart. But if the sister who moves in the big swings will learn from the other to be careful in details, and if the smaller mind will allow itself to be enlarged by learning from the habitually broader view of the other, each will grow in proportion, and two women who began life as enemies in temperament can end it as happy friends.

There are similar cases of brothers who clash, but they are not so evident, for when men do not agree they leave one another alone. Women do not seem to be able to do that. It is good to leave one another alone when there is the clashing tendency, but it is better to conquer the clashing and learn to agree.

So long as the normal course of my life leads me to live with some one who rubs me the wrong way I am not free until I have learned to live with that some one in quiet content. I never gain my freedom by running away. The bondage is in me always, so long as the other person's presence can rouse it. The only way is to fight it out inside of one's self. When we can get the co-operation of the other so much the better. But no one's co-operation is necessary for us to find our own freedom, and with it an intelligent, tolerant kindliness.

"Mother, you take that seat. No, not that one, Mother—the sun comes in that window. Children, move aside and let your grandmother get to her seat."

The young woman was very much in earnest in seeing that her mother had a comfortable seat, that she had not the discomfort of the hot sun, that the children made way for her so that she could move into her seat comfortably. All her words were thoughtful and courteous, but the spirit and the tone of her words were quite the reverse of courteous. If some listener with his eyes shut had heard the tone without understanding the words he might easily have thought that the woman was talking to a little dog.

Poor "Mother" trotted into her seat with the air of a little dog who was so well trained that he did at once what his mistress ordered. It was very evident that "Mother's" will had been squeezed out of her and trampled upon for years by her dutiful daughter, who looked out always that "Mother" had the best, without the first scrap of respect for "Mother's" free, human soul.

The grandchildren took the spirit of their mother's words rather than the words themselves, and treated their grandmother as if she were a sort of traveling idiot tagged on to them, to whom they had to be decently respectful whenever their mother's eye was upon them, and whom they ignored entirely when their mother looked the other way.

It so happened that I was sitting next to this particular mother who had been poked into a comfortable seat by her careful daughter. And, after a number of other suggestions had been poked at her with a view to adding to her comfort, she turned to me and in a quaint, confidential way, with the gentle voice of a habitual martyr, and at the same time a twinkle of humor in her eye, she said "They think, you know, I don't know anything."

And after that we had a little talk about matters of the day which proved to me that "Mother" had a mind broader and certainly more quiet than her daughter. I studied the daughter with interest after knowing "Mother" better, and her habitual strain of voice and manner were pathetic. By making a care of her mother instead of a companion, she was not only guilty of disrespect to a soul which, however weak it may have been in allowing itself to be directed in all minor matters, had its own firm principles which were not overridden nor even disturbed by the daughter's dominance. If the daughter had only dropped her strain of care and her habit of "bossing" she would have found a true companion in her mother, and would have been a healthier and happier woman herself.

In pleasant contrast to this is the story of a family which had an old father who had lost his mind entirely, and had grown decrepit and childish in the extreme. The sons and daughters tended him like a baby and loved him with gentle, tender respect. There was no embarrassment for his loss of mind, no thought of being distressed or pained by it, and because his children took their father's state so quietly and without shame, every guest who came took it in the same way, and there was no thought of keeping the father out of sight. He sat in the living-room in his comfortable chair, and always one child or another was sitting right beside him with a smiling face. Instead of being a trying member of the family, as happens in so many cases, this old father seemed to bring content and rest to his children through their loving care for him.

Very often—I might almost say always—the trying member of the family is trying only because we make her so by our attitude toward her, let her be grandmother, mother, or maiden aunt. Even the proverbial mother-in-law grows less difficult as our attitude toward her is relieved of the strain of detesting everything she does, and expecting to detest everything that she is going to do. With every trying friend we have, if we yield to him in all minor matters we find the settling of essential questions wonderfully less difficult.

A son had a temper and the girl he married had a temper. The mother loved her son with the selfish love with which so many mothers burden their children, and thought that he alone of all men had a right to lose his temper. Consequently she excused her son and blamed her daughter-in-law. If there were a mild cyclone roused between the two married people the son would turn to his mother to hear what a martyr he was and what misfortune he had to bear in having been so easily mistaken in the woman he married. Thus the mother-in-law, who felt that she was protecting her poor son, was really breeding dissension between two people who could have been the best possible friends all their lives.

The young wife very soon became ashamed of her temper and worked until she conquered it, but it was not until her mother-in-law had been out of this world for years that her husband discovered what he had lost in turning away from his wife's friendship, and it was only by the happy accident of severe illness that he ever discovered his mistake at all, and gained freedom from the bondage of his own temper enough to appreciate his wife.

If, however, the wife had yielded in the beginning not only to her husband's bad temper but also to the antagonism of her mother-in-law, which was, of course, annoying in many petty ways, she might have gained her husband's friendship, and it is possible that she might, moreover, have gained the friendship of her mother-in-law.

The best rule with regard to all trying members of the family is to yield to them always in non-essentials; and when you disagree in essentials stick to the principle which you believe to be right, but stick to it without resistance. Believe your way, but make yourself willing that the trying member should believe her way. Make an opportunity of what appears to be a limitation, and, believe me, your trying member can become a blessing to you.

I go further than that—I truly believe that to make the best of life every family should have a trying member. When we have no trying member of our family, and life goes along smoothly, as a matter of course, the harmony is very liable to be spurious, and a sudden test will all at once knock such a family into discord, much to the surprise of every member. When we go through discord to harmony, and once get into step, we are very likely to keep in step:

Be willing, then, make yourself willing, that the trying member should be in the way. Hope that she will stay in your family until you have succeeded in dropping not only all resistance to her being there, but every resistance to her various ways in detail. Bring her annoying ways up to your mind voluntarily when you are away from her. If you do that you will find all the resistances come with them and you can relax out of the strain then and there. You will find that when you get home or come down to breakfast in the morning (for many resistances are voluntarily thrown off in the night) you will have a pleasanter feeling toward the trying member, and it comes so spontaneously that you will be surprised yourself at the absence of the strain of resistance in you.

Believe me when I say this: the yielding in the non-essentials, singularly enough, gives one strength to refuse to yield in principles. But we must always remember that if we want to find real peace, while we refuse to yield in our own principles so long as we believe them to be true, we must be entirely willing that others should differ from us in belief.

CHAPTER VI

Irritable Husbands

SUPPOSE your husband got impatient and annoyed with you because you did not seem to enter heartily into the interests of his work and sympathize with its cares and responsibilities and soothe him out of the nervous harassments. Would you not perhaps feel a little sore that he seemed to expect all from you and to give nothing in return? I know how many women will say that is all very well, but the husband and father should feel as much interest in the home and the children as the wife and mother does. That is, of course, true up to a certain point, always in general, and when his help is really necessary in particular. But a man cannot enter into the details of his wife's duties at home any more than a woman can enter into the details of her husband's duties at his office.

Then, again, my readers may say: "But a woman's nervous system is more sensitive than a man's; she needs help and consolation. She needs to have some one on whom she can lean." Now the answer to that will probably be surprising, but an intelligent understanding and comprehension of it would make a very radical difference in the lives of many men and women who have agreed to live together for life—for better and for worse.

Now the truth is man's nervous system is quite as sensitive as a woman's, but the woman's temptation to emotion makes her appear more sensitive, and her failure to control her emotions ultimately increases the sensitiveness of her nerves so that they are more abnormal than her husband's. Even that is not always true The other day a woman sat in tears and distress telling of the hardness of heart, the restlessness, the irritability, the thoughtlessness, the unkindness of her husband. Her face was drawn with suffering. She insisted that she was not complaining, that it was her deep and tender love for her husband that made her suffer so. "But it is killing me, it is killing me," she said, and one who saw her could well believe it. And if the distress and the great strain upon her nerves had kept on it certainly would have made her ill, if not have actually ended her life with a nervous collapse.

The friend in whom she confided sat quietly and heard her through. She let her pour herself out to the very finish until she stopped because there was nothing more to say. Then, by means of a series of gentle, well-adapted questions, she drew from the wife a recognition—for the first time—of the fact that she really did nothing whatever for her husband and expected him to do everything for her. Perhaps she put on a pretty dress for him in order to look attractive when he came home, but if he did not notice how well she looked, and was irritable about something in the house, she would be dissolved in tears because she had not proved attractive and pleased him. Maybe she had tried to have a dinner that he especially liked; then if he did not notice the food, and seemed distracted about something that was worrying him, she would again be dissolved in tears because he "appreciated nothing that she tried to do for him."

Now it is perfectly true that this husband was irritable and brutal; he had no more consideration for his wife than he had for any one else. But his wife was doing all in her power to fan his irritability into flame and to increase his brutality. She was attitudinizing in her own mind as a martyr. She was demanding kindness and attention and sympathy from her husband, and because she demanded it she never got it.

A woman can demand without demanding imperiously. There is more selfish demanding in a woman's emotional suffering because her husband does not do this or that or the other for her sake than there is in a tornado of man's irritability or anger. You see, a woman's demanding spirit is covered with the mush of her emotions. A man's demanding spirit stands out in all its naked ugliness. One is just as bad as the other. One is just as repulsive as the other.

It is a radical, practical impossibility to bring loving-kindness out of any one by demanding it. Loving-kindness, thoughtfulness, and consideration have got to be born spontaneously in a man's own mind to be anything at all, and no amount of demanding on the part of his wife can force it.

When this little lady of whom I have been writing found that she had been demanding from her husband what he really ought to have given her as a matter of course, and that she had used up all her strength in suffering because he did not give it, and had used none of her strength in the effort to be patient and quiet in waiting for him to come to his senses, she went home and began a new life. She was a plucky little woman and very intelligent when once her eyes were opened. She recognized the fact that her suffering was resistance to her husband's irritable selfishness, and she stopped resisting.

It was a long and hard struggle of days, weeks, and months, but it brought a very happy reward. When a man is irritable and ugly, and his wife offers no resistance either in anger or suffering, the irritability and ugliness react upon himself, and if there is something better in him he begins to perceive the irritability in its true colors. That is what happened to this man. As his wife stopped demanding he began to give. As his wife's nerves became calm and quiet his nerves quieted and calmed. Finally his wife discovered that much of his irritability had been roused through nervous anxiety in regard to his business about which he had told her nothing whatever because it "was not his way."

There is nothing in the world that so strengthens nerves as the steady use of the will to drop resistance and useless emotions and get a quiet control. This woman gained that strength, and to her surprise one day her husband turned to her with a full account of all his business troubles and she met his mind quietly, as one business man might meet another, and without in the least expressing her pleasure or her surprise. She took all the good change in him as a matter of course.

Finally one day it came naturally and easily to talk over the past. She found that her husband from day to day had dreaded coming home. The truth was that he had dreaded his own irritability as much as he had dreaded her emotional demanding. But he did not know it—he did not know what was the matter at all. He simply knew vaguely that he was a brute, that he felt like a brute, and that he did not know how to stop being a brute. His wife knew that he was a brute, and at the same time she felt throughly convinced that she was a suffering martyr. He was dreading to come home and she was dreading to have him come home—and there they were in a continuous nightmare. Now they have left the nightmare far, far behind, and each one knows that the other has one good friend in the world in whom he or she can feel entire confidence, and their friendship is growing stronger and clearer and more normal every day.

It is not the ceremony that makes the marriage: the ceremony only begins it. Marriage is a slow and careful adjustment. A true story which illustrates the opposite of this condition is that of a man and woman who were to all appearances happily married for years. They were apparently the very closest friends. The man's nerves were excitable and peculiar, and his wife adjusted herself to them by indulging them and working in every way to save him from friction. No woman could stand that constant work of adjustment which was in reality maladjustment, and this wife's nerves broke down unexpectedly and completely.

When our nerves get weak we are unable to repress resistance which in a stronger state we had covered up. This wife, while she had indulged and protected her husband's peculiarities, had subconsciously resisted them. When she became ill her subconscious resistance came to the surface. She surprised herself by growing impatient with her husband. He, of course; retorted. As she grew worse he did not find his usual comfort from her care, and instead of trying to help her to get well he turned his back on her and complained to another woman. Finally the friction of the two nervous systems became dangerously intense. Each was equally obstinate, and there was nothing to do but to separate The woman died of a broken heart, and the man is probably insane for the rest of his life.

It was nothing but the mismanagement of their own and each other's nerves that made all this terrible trouble. Their love seemed genuine at first, and could certainly have grown to be really genuine if they had become truly adjusted. And the saddest part of the whole story is that they were both peculiarly adapted to be of use to their fellow-men. During the first years of their life their home was a delight to all their friends.

Tired nerves are likely to close up a man or make him irritable, complaining, and ugly, whereas the tendency in a woman is to be irritable, complaining, and tearful. Now of course when each one is selfishly looking out for his or her comfort neither one can be expected to understand the other. The man thinks he is entirely justified in being annoyed with the woman's tearful, irritable complaints, and so he is—in a way. The woman thinks that she has a right to suffer because of her husband's irritable ugliness, and so she has—in a way. But in the truest way, and the way which appeals to every one's common sense, neither one has a right to complain of the other, and each one by right should have first made things better and clearer in himself and herself.

Human nature is not so bad—really in its essence it is not bad at all. If we only give the other man a real chance. It is the pushing and pulling and demanding of one human being toward another that smother the best in us, and make life a fearful strain. Of course there is a healthy demanding as well as an unhealthy demanding, but, so far as I know, the healthy demanding can come only when we are clear of personal resistance and can demand on the strength of a true principle and without selfish emotion. There is a kind of gentle, motherly contempt with which some women speak of their husbands, which must get on a man's nerves very painfully. It is intensely and most acutely annoying. And yet I have heard good women speak in that way over and over again. The gentleness and motherliness are of course neither of them real in such cases. The gentle, motherly tone is used to cover up their own sense of superiority.

"Poor boy, poor boy," they may say; "a man is really like a child." So he may be—so he often is childish, and sometimes childish in the extreme. But where could you find greater and more abject childishness than in a woman's ungoverned emotions?

A woman must respect the manliness of her husband's soul, and must cling to her belief in its living existence behind any amount of selfish, restless irritability, if she is going to find a friend in him or be a friend to him. She must also know that his nervous system may be just as sensitive as hers. Sometimes it is more sensitive, and should be accordingly respected. Demand nothing and expect nothing, but hold him to his best in your mind and wait.

That is a rule that would work wonderfully if every woman who is puzzled about her husband's restlessness and lack of interest in home affairs would apply it steadily and for long enough. It is impossible to manufacture a happy, sympathetic married life artificially—impossible! But as each one looks to one's self and does one's part fully, and then is willing to wait for the other, the happiness and the sympathy, the better power for work and the joyful ability to play come—they do come; they are real and alive and waiting for us as we get clear from the interferences.

"Why doesn't my husband like to stay with me when he comes home? Why can't we have nice, cozy times together?" a wife asks with sad longing in her eyes.

And to the same friend the husband (who is, by the way, something of a pig) says: "I should be glad to stay with Nellie often in the evening, but she will always talk about her worries, and she worries about the family in a way that is idiotic. She is always sure that George will catch the measles because a boy in the next street has them, and she is always sure that our children do not have the advantages nor the good manners that other children have. If it is not one thing it is another; whenever we are alone there is something to complain of, and her last complaint was about her own selfishness." Then he laughed at what he considered a good joke, and in five minutes had forgotten all about her.

This wife, in a weak, selfish little way, was trying to give her husband her confidence, and her complaint about her own selfishness was genuine. She wanted his help to get out of it. If he had given her just a little gracious attention and told her how impossible it was really to discuss the children when she began the conversation with whining complaint, she would have allowed herself to be taught and their intercourse would have improved. On the other hand, if the wife had realized that her husband came home from the cares of his business tired and nervous, and if she had talked lightly and easily on general subjects and tried to follow his interests, when his nerves were rested and quiet she might have found him ready and able to give her a little lift with regard to the children.

It is interesting and it is delightful to see how, as we each work first to bear our own burdens, we not only find ourselves ready and able to lighten the burdens of others but find others who are helpful to us.

A woman who finds her husband "so restless and irritable" should remember that in reality a man's nervous system is just as sensitive as a woman's, and, with a steady and consistent effort to bear her own burdens and to work out her own problems, should prepare herself to lighten her husband's burdens and help to solve his problems; that is the truest way of bringing him to the place where he will be glad to share her burdens with her as well as his own.

But we want to remember that there is a radical difference between indulging another's selfishness, and waiting, with patient yielding, for him to discover his selfishness himself, and to act unselfishly from his own free will.

CHAPTER VII

Quiet vs. Chronic Excitement

SOME women live in a chronic state of excitement all the time and they do not find it out until they get ill. Even then they do not always find it out, and then they get more ill.

It is really much the same with excitable women as with a man who thinks he must always keep a little stimulant in himself in order to keep about his work. When a bad habit is established in us we feel unnatural if we give the habit up for a moment—and we feel natural when we are in it—but it is poison all the same.

If a woman has a habit of constantly snuffing or clearing her throat, or rocking a rocking chair, or chattering to whoever may be near her she would feel unnatural and weird if she were suddenly wrenched out of any of these things. And yet the poisoning process goes on just the same.

When it seems immaterial to us that we should be natural we are in a pretty bad way and the worst of it is we do not know it.

I once took a friend with me into the country who was one of those women who lived on excitement in every-day life. When she dressed in the morning she dressed in excitement. She went down to breakfast in excitement. She went about the most humdrum everyday affairs excited. Every event in life—little or big—was an excitement to her—and she went to bed tired out with excitement—over nothing.

We went deep in the woods and in the mountains, full of great powerful quiet.

When my friend first got there she was excited about her arrival, she was excited about the house and the people in it, but in the middle of the night she jumped up in bed with a groan of torture.

I thought she had been suddenly taken ill and started up quickly from my end of the room to see what was the trouble.

"Oh, oh," she groaned, "the quiet! It is so quiet!" Her brain which had been in a whirl of petty excitement felt keen pain when the normal quiet touched it.

Fortunately this woman had common sense and I could gradually explain the truth to her, and she acted upon it and got rested and strong and quiet.

I knew another woman who had been wearing shoes that were too tight for her and that pinched her toes all together. The first time she wore shoes that gave her feet room enough the muscles of her feet hurt her so that she could hardly walk.

Of course, having been cramped into abnormal contraction the process of expanding to freedom would be painful.

If you had held your fist clenched tight for years, or months, or even weeks, how it would hurt to open it so that you could have free use of your fingers.

The same truth holds good with a fist that has been clenched, a foot that has been pinched, or a brain that has been contracted with excitement.

The process leading from the abnormal to the normal is always a painful one. To stay in the abnormal means blindness, constantly limiting power and death.

To come out into a normal atmosphere and into a normal way of living means clearer sight, constantly increasing power, and fresh life.

This habit of excitement is not only contracting to the brain; it has its effect over the whole body. If there is any organ that is weaker than any other the excitement eventually shows itself. A woman may be suffering from indigestion, or she may be running up large doctor's bills because of either one of a dozen other organic disturbances, with no suspicion that the cause of the whole trouble is that the noisy, excited, strained habits of her life have robbed her body of the vitality it needed to keep it in good running order.

As if an engineer threw his coal all over the road and having no fuel for his engine wondered that it would not run. Stupid women we are—most of us!

The trouble is that many of us are so deeply immersed in the habit of excitement that we do not know it.

It is a healthy thing to test ourselves and to really try to find ourselves out. It is not only healthy; it is deeply interesting.

If quiet of the woods, or, any other quiet place, makes us fidgety, we may be sure that our own state is abnormal and we had better go into the woods as often as possible until we feel ourselves to be a part of the quiet there.

If we go into the woods and get soothed and quieted and then come out and get fussed up and excited so that we feel painfully the contrast between the quiet and our every-day life, then we can know that we are living in the habit of abnormal excitement and we can set to work to stop it.

"That is all very well," I hear my readers say, "but how are you going to stop living in abnormal excitement when every circumstance and every person about you is full of it and knows nothing else?"

If you really want to do it and would feel interested to make persistent effort I can give you the recipe and I can promise any woman that if she perseveres until she has found the way she will never cease to be grateful.

If you start with the intention of taking the five minutes' search for quiet every day, do not let your intention be weakened or yourself discouraged if for some days you see no result at all.

At first it may be that whatever quiet you find will seem so strange that it will annoy you or make you very nervous, but if you persist and work right through, the reward will be worth the pains many times over.

Sometimes quieting our minds helps us to quiet our bodies; sometimes we must quiet our bodies first before we can find the way to a really quiet mind. The attention of the mind to quiet the body, of course, reacts back on to the mind, and from there we can pass on to thinking quietly. Each individual must judge for herself as to the best way of reaching the quiet. I will give several recipes and you can take your choice.

First, to quiet the body:—

1. Lie still and see how quietly you can breathe.

2. Sit still and let your head droop very slowly forward until finally it hangs down with its whole weight. Then lift it up very, very slowly and feel as if you pushed it all the way up from the lower part of your spine, or, better still, as if it grew up, so that you feel the slow, creeping, soothing motion all the way up your spine while your head is coming up, and do not let your head come to an entirely erect

position until your chest is as high as you can hold it comfortably. When your head is erect take a long, quiet breath and drop it again. You can probably drop it and raise it twice in the five minutes. Later on it should take the whole five minutes to drop it and raise it once and an extra two minutes for the long breath.

When you have dropped your head as far as you can, pause for a full minute without moving at all and feel heavy; then begin at the lower part of your spine and very slowly start to raise it. Be careful not to hold your breath, and watch to breathe as easily and quietly as you can while your head is moving.

If this exercise hurts the back of your neck or any part of your spine, don't be troubled by it, but go right ahead and you will soon come to where it not only does not hurt, but is very restful.

When you have reached an erect position again stay there quietly—first take long gentle breaths and let them get shorter and shorter until they are a good natural length, then forget your breathing altogether and sit still as if you never had moved, you never were going to move, and you never wanted to move.

This emphasizes the good natural quiet in your brain and so makes you more sensitive to unquiet.

Gradually you will get the habit of catching yourself in states of unnecessary excitement; at such times you cannot go off by yourself and go through the exercises. You cannot even stop where you are and go through them, but you can recall the impression made on your brain at the time you did them and in that way rule out your excitement and gain the real power that should be in its place.

So little by little the state of excitement becomes as unpleasant as a cloud of dust on a windy day and the quiet is as pleasant as under the trees on top of a hill in the best kind of a June day.

The trouble is so many of us live in a cloud of dust that we do not suspect even the existence of the June day, but if we are fortunate enough once or twice even to get to sneezing from the dust, and so to recognize its unpleasantness, then we want to look carefully to see if there is not a way out of it.

It is then that we can get the beginning of the real quiet which is the normal atmosphere of every human being.

But we must persist for a long time before we can feel established in the quiet itself. What is worth having is worth working for—and the more it is worth having, the harder work is required to get it.

Nerves form habits, and our nerves not only get the habit of living in the dust, but the nerves of all about us have the same habit. So that when at first we begin to get into clear air, we may almost dislike it, and rush back into the dust again, because we and our friends are accustomed to it.

All that bad habit has to be fought, and conquered, and there are many difficulties in the way of persistence, but the reward is worth it all, as I hope to show in later articles.

I remember once walking in a crowded street where the people were hurrying and rushing, where every one's face was drawn and knotted, and nobody seemed to be having a good time. Suddenly and unexpectedly I saw a man coming toward me with a face so quiet that it showed out like a little bit of calm in a tornado. He looked like a common, everyday man of the world, so far as his dress and general bearing went, and his features were not at all unusual, but his expression was so full of quiet interest as to be the greatest contrast to those about him. He was not thinking his own thoughts either—he was one of the crowd and a busy, interested observer.

He might have said, "You silly geese, what are you making all this fuss about, you can do it much better if you will go more easily." If that was his thought it came from a very kindly sense of humor, and he gave me a new realization of what it meant, practically, to be in the world and not of it.

If you are in the world you can live, and observe, and take a much better part in its workings. If you are of it, you are simply whirled in an eddy of dust, however you may pose to yourself or to others.

CHAPTER VIII

The Tired Emphasis

"I AM so tired, so tired—I go to bed tired, I get up tired, and I am tired all the time."

How many women—how many hundred women, how many thousand women—say that to themselves and to others constantly.

It is perfectly true; they are tired all the time; they do go to bed tired and get up tired and stay tired all day.

If, however, they could only know how very much they increase their fatigue by their constant mental emphasis of it, and if at the same time they could turn their wills in the direction of decreasing the fatigue, instead of emphasizing it, a very large percentage of the tired feeling could be done away with altogether.

Many women would gladly make more of an effort in the direction of rest if they knew how, and I propose in this article to give a prescription for the cure of the tired emphasis which, if followed, will bring happy results.

When you go to bed at night, no matter how tired you feel, instead of thinking how tired you are, think how good it is that you can go to bed to get rested.

It will probably seem absurd to you at first. You may say to yourself: "How ridiculous, going to bed to get rested, when I have only one short night to rest in, and one or two weeks in bed would not rest me thoroughly."

The answer to that is that if you have only one night in which to rest, you want to make the most of that night, and if you carry the tired emphasis to bed with you you are really holding on to the tired.

This is as practically true as if you stepped into a bog and then sat in it and looked forlorn and said. "What a terrible thing it is that I should be in a bog like this; just think of having to sit in a black, muddy bog all the time," and staying there you made no effort whatever to get out of it, even though there was dry land right in front of you.

Again you may answer: "But in my tired bog there is no dry land in front of me, none at all."

I say to that, there is much more dry land than you think—if you will open your eyes—and to open your eyes you must make an effort.

No one knows, who has not tried, what a good strong effort will do in the right direction, when we have been living and slipping back in the wrong direction.

The results of such efforts seem at times wonderful to those who have learned the right direction for the first time.

To get rid of the tired emphasis when we have been fixed in it, a very strong effort is necessary at first, and gradually it gets easier, and easier, until we have cast off the tired emphasis entirely and have the habit of looking toward rest.

We must say to ourselves with decision in so many words, and must think the meaning of the words and insist upon it: "I am very tired. Yes, of course, I am very tired, but I am going to bed to get rested."

There are a hundred little individual ways that we can talk to ourselves, and turn ourselves toward rest, at the end of the day when the time comes to rest.

One way to begin, which is necessary to most of us, is to stop resisting the tired. Every complaint of fatigue, whether it is merely in our own minds, or is made to others, is full of resistance, and resistance to any sort of fatigue emphasizes it proportionately.

That is why it is good to say to ourselves: "Yes, I am tired; I am awfully tired. I am willing to be tired."

When we have used our wills to drop the nervous and muscular contractions that the fatigue has caused, we can add with more emphasis and more meaning, "and I am going to bed to get rested."

Some one could say just here: "That is all very well for an ordinarily tired person, but it would never do me any good. I am too tired even to try it."

The answer to that is, the more tired you are, the more you need to try it, and the more interesting the experiment will be.

Also the very effort of your brain needed to cast off the tired emphasis will be new to you, and thought in a new direction is always restful in itself. Having learned to cast off the tired emphasis when we go to bed at night, we can gradually learn to cast it off before we go to meals, and at odd opportunities throughout the day.

The more tired we are, the more we need to minimize our fatigue by the intelligent use of our own wills.

Who cares for a game that is simple and easy? Who cares for a game when you beat as a matter of course, and without any effort on your part at all?

Whoever cares for games at all cares most for good, stiff ones, where, when you have beaten, you can feel that you have really accomplished something; and when you have not beaten, you have at least learned points that will enable you to beat the next time, or the next to the next time—or sometime. And everyone who really loves a game wants to stick to it until he has conquered and is proficient.

Why not wake up, and realize that same interest and courage in this biggest game of all—this game of life?

We must play it!

Few of us are cowards enough to put ourselves out of it. Unless we play it and obey the rules we do not really play at all.

Many of us do not know the rules, but it is our place to look about and find them out.

Many more of us think that we can play the game better if we make up rules of our own, and leave out whatever regular rules we do know, that do not suit our convenience.

But that never works.

It only sometimes seems to work; and although plain common sense shows us over and over that the game played according to our own ideas amounts to nothing, it is strange to see how many work and push to play the game in their own way instead of in the game's way.

It is strange to see how many shove blindly in this direction, and that direction, to cut their way through a jungle, when there is the path just by them, if they will take it.

Most of us do not know our own power because we would rather stay in a ditch and complain.

Strength begets strength, and we can only find our greater power, by using intelligently, and steadily, the power we have.

CHAPTER IX

How to be Ill and get Well

ILLNESS seems to be one of the hardest things to happen to a busy woman. Especially hard is it when a woman must live from hand to mouth, and so much illness means, almost literally, so much less food.

Sometimes one is taken so suddenly and seriously ill that it is impossible to think of whether one has food and shelter or not; one must just be taken care of or die. It does not seem to matter which at the time.

Then another must meet the difficulty. It is the little nagging illnesses that make the trouble—just enough to keep a woman at home a week or ten days or more, and deprive her of wages which she might have been receiving, and which she very much needs.

These are the illnesses that are hard to bear.

Many a woman has suffered through an illness like this, which has dragged out from day to day, and finally left her pale and weak, to return to her work with much less strength than she needs for what is before her.

After forcing herself to work day after day, her strength comes back so slowly, that she appears to go through another illness, on her feet, and "in the harness," before she can really call herself well again.

There are a few clear points which, if intelligently comprehended, could teach one how to meet an illness, and if persistently acted upon, would not only shorten it, but would lighten the convalescence so that when the invalid returned to her work she would feel stronger than before she was taken ill.

When one is taken with a petty illness, if it is met in an intelligent way, the result can be a good rest, and one feels much better, and has a more healthy appearance, than before the attack.

This effect has been so often experienced that with some people there is a little bit of pleasantry passed on meeting a friend, in the remark: "Why, how do you do; how well you look—you must have been ill!"

If we remember when we are taken ill that nature always tends towards health, we will study carefully to fulfill nature's conditions in order to cure the disease.

We will rest quietly, until nature in her process toward health has reached health. In that way our illness can be the means of giving us a good rest, and, while we may feel the loss of the energy of which the disease has robbed us, we also feel the good effects of the rest which we have given to organs which were only tired.

These organs which have gained rest can, in their turn, help toward renewing the strength of the organs which had been out of order, and thus we get up from an illness looking so well, and feeling so well, that we do not regret the loss of time, and feel ready to work, and to gradually make up the loss of money.

Of course, the question is, how to fulfill the conditions so that this happy result can be attained.

In the first place, *do not fret.*

"But how can I help fretting?" someone will say, "when I am losing money every day, and do not know how many more days I may be laid up?"

The answer to that is: "If you will think of the common sense of it, you can easily see that the strain of fretting is interfering radically with your getting well. For when you are using up strength to fret, you are simply robbing yourself of the vitality which would be used directly in the cure of your illness."

Not only that, but the strain of fretting increases the strain of illness, and is not only preventing you from getting well, but it is tending to keep you ill.

When we realize that fact, it seems as if it would be an easy matter to stop fretting in order to get well.

It is as senseless to fret about an illness, no matter how much just cause we may feel we have, as it would be to walk west when our destination was directly east.

Stop and think of it. Is not that true? Imagine a child with a pin pricking him, kicking, and screaming, and squirming with the pain, so that his mother—try as carefully as she may—takes five minutes to find the pin and get it out, when she might have done it and relieved him in five seconds, if only the child had kept still and let her.

So it is with us when Mother Nature is working with wise steadiness to find the pin that is making us ill, and to get it out. We fret and worry so that it takes her ten or twenty days to do the good work that she might have done in three.

In order to drop the fretting, we must use our wills to think, and feel, and act, so that the way may be opened for health to come to us in the quickest possible time.

Every contraction of worry which appears in the muscles we must drop, so that we lie still with a sense of resting, and waiting for the healing power, which is surely working within us, to make us well.

We can do this by a deliberate use of our wills.

If we could take our choice between medicine, and the curative power of dropping anxiety and letting ourselves get well, there would be no hesitancy, provided we understood the alternatives.

I speak of fretting first because it is so often the strongest interference with health.

Defective circulation is the trouble in most diseases, and we should do all we can to open the channels so that the circulation, being free elsewhere, can tend to open the way to greater freedom in the part diseased. The contractions caused by fretting impede the circulation still more, and therefore heighten the disease.

If once, by a strong use of the will, we drop the fretting and give ourselves up entirely to letting nature cure us, then we can study, with interest, to fulfill other necessary conditions. We can give ourselves the right amount of fresh air, of nourishment, of bathing, and the right sort of medicine, if any is needed.

Thus, instead of interfering with nature, we are doing all in our power to aid her; and when nature and the invalid work in harmony, health comes on apace.

When illness brings much pain and discomfort with it, the endeavor to relax out of the contractions caused by the pain, are of the same service as dropping contractions caused by the fretting.

If one can find a truly wise doctor, or nurse, in such an illness as I refer to, get full instructions in just one visit, and then follow those directions explicitly, only one visit will be needed, probably, and the gain from that will pay for it many times over.

This article is addressed especially to those who are now in health.

It is perhaps too much to expect one in the midst of an illness to start at once with what we may call the curative attitude, although it could be done, but if those who are now well and strong will read and get a good understanding of this healthy way of facing an illness, and get it into their subconscious minds, they will find that if at any time they should be unfortunate enough to be attacked with illness, they can use the knowledge to very real advantage, and—what is more—they can, with the right tact, help others to use it also.

To see the common sense of a process and, when we have not the opportunity to use the laws ourselves, to help others by means of our knowledge, impresses our own brains more thoroughly with the truth, especially if our advice is taken and acted upon and thus proved to be true.

It must not be forgotten, however, that to help another man or woman to a healthy process of getting well requires gentle patience and quiet, steady, unremitting tact.

CHAPTER X

Is Physical Culture good for Girls?

A NUMBER of women were watching a game of basket-ball played by some high-school girls. In the interim for rest one woman said to her neighbor: "Do you see that girl flat on her back, looking like a very heavy bag of sand?"

"Yes," the answer was; "what under the sun is she doing that for? She looks heavy and lazy and logy, while the other girls are talking and laughing and having a good time."

"You wait and watch her play," responded the first woman. And so they waited and watched, and to the astonishment of the friend the girl who had looked "lazy and logy," lying flat on her back during the rest-time, was the most active of the players, and really saved the game.

When the game was finished the woman said to her friend with surprise in her voice: "How did you see through that, and understand what that girl was aiming for?"

The answer was: "Well, I know the girl, and both she and I have read Kipling's 'The Maltese Cat.' Don't you remember how the best polo ponies in that story, when they were off duty, hung their heads and actually made themselves looked fagged, in order to be fresher when the time came to play? And how 'The Maltese Cat' scouted the silly ponies who held their heads up and kicked and looked alert while they waited? And don't you remember the result?"

"No, I never read the story, but I have certainly seen your point prove itself to-day. I shall read it at once. Meanwhile, I want to speak to that clever girl who could catch a point like that and use it."

"Take care, please, that you do not mention it to her at all," said the friend. "You will draw her attention back to herself and likely as not make her lose the next game. Points like that have got to be worked on without self-consciousness, not talked about."

And so the women told the child they were glad that her side won the game and never mentioned her own part in it at all. After all she had only found the law that the more passive you can be when it is time to rest, the more alert you are and the more powerful in activity. The polo pony knew it as a matter of course. We humans have to discover it.

Let us, just for the interest of it, follow that same basket-ball player a little more closely. Was she well developed and evenly trained in her muscles? Yes, very. Did she go to gymnasium, or did she scorn it? She went, twice a week regularly, and had good fun there; but there was just this contrast between her and most of the girls in the class: Jane, as we will call her, went to gymnasium as a means to an end. She found that she got an even development there which enabled her to walk better, to play better, and to work better. In gymnasium she laid her muscular foundation on which to build all the good, active work of her life. The gymnasium she went to, however, was managed in an unusual way except for the chest weights, which always "opened the ball," the members of the class never knew what work they were to do. Their minds were kept alert throughout the hour and a half. If their attention wavered they tripped or got behind in the exercise, and the mental action which went into the movement of every muscle made the body alive with the healthy activity of a well-concentrated, well-directed mind.

Another point which our young friend learned at gymnasium was to direct her mind only on to the muscles that were needed. Did you ever try to clench your fist so tight that it could not be opened? If not, try it, and relax all over your body while you are keeping your fist tight closed. You will see that the more limp your body becomes the tighter you can keep your fist clenched. All the force goes in that one direction. In this way a moderately strong girl can keep a strong man hard at work for several minutes before he can make any impression on the closed hand. That illustrates in a simple way the fact that the most wholesome concentration is that which comes from dropping everything that interferes—letting the force of mind or body flow only in the direction in which it is to be used.

Many girls use their brains in the wrong way while on the gymnasium floor by saying to themselves, "I cannot do that." The brain is so full of that thought that the impression an open brain would receive has no chance to enter, and the result is an awkward, nervous, and uncertain movement. If a girl's brain and muscle were so relaxed that the impression on the one would cause a correct use and movement of the other how easy it would be thereafter to apply the proper tension to the muscle at the proper time without overtaxing the nerves.

Some one has well said that "it is training, not straining, that we want in our gymnasiums." Only when a girl is trained from this point of view does she get real training.

This basket-ball player had also been taught how to rest after exercise in a way which appealed to her especially, because of her interest which had already been aroused in Kipling's polo pony. She was taught intelligently that if, after vigorous exercise, when the blood is coursing rapidly all over the body, you allow yourself to be entirely open and passive, the blood finds no interruptions in its work and can carry away the waste matter much more effectually. In that way you get the full result of the exercise. It is not necessary always to lie down to have your body passive enough after vigorous exercise to get the best results. If you sit down after exercise you want to sit without tension. Or if you walk home from gymnasium you want to walk loosely and freely, keeping your chest up and a little in advance, and pushing with the ball of your back foot with a good, rhythmic balance. As this is the best way to sit and the best way to walk—gymnasium or no gymnasium—to look out for a well-balanced sitting and a well-balanced walk directly after vigorous exercise, keeps us in good form for sitting and walking all the time.

I know of a professor in one of our large colleges who was offered also a professorship in a woman's college, and he refused to accept because he said women's minds did not react. When he lectured to girls he found that, however attentively they might seem to listen, there was no response. They gave nothing in return.

Of course this is not true of all girls, and of course the gentleman who refused the chair in the woman's college would agree that it is not true of all girls, but if those who read the anecdote would, instead of getting indignant, just look into the matter a little, they would see how true it is of many girls, and by thinking a little further we can see that it is not at present the girls' fault. A hundred years ago girls were not expected to think. I remember an anecdote which a very intelligent old lady used to tell me about her mother. Once, when she was a little girl, her mother found some fault with her which the daughter knew to be unjust, and she answered timidly, "But, Mother, I think—"

"Abigail," came the sharp reminder, "you've no business to think."

One hundred years ago it was only the very exceptional girls who really thought. Now we are gradually working toward the place where every girl will think. And surely it cannot be very long now before the united minds of a class of college girls will have the habit of reacting so that any man will feel in his own brain a vigorous result from lecturing to them.

This fact that a girl's brain does not react is proved in many ways. Most of the women who come to nerve specialists seem to feel that they are to sit still and be cured, while the men who come respond and do their part much more intelligently—the result being that men get out of "nerves" in half the time and stay out, whereas girls often get out a little way and slump (literally slump) back again before they can be helped to respond truly enough to get well and keep themselves well. This information is given only with an idea of stirring girls up to their best possibilities, for there is not a woman born with a sound mind who is not capable of reacting mentally, in a greater or less degree, to all that she hears, provided she uses her will consciously to form the new habit.

Now this need of intelligent reaction is just the trouble with girls and physical culture. Physical culture should be a means to an end—and that is all, absolutely all. It is delightful and strengthening when it is taught thoughtfully as a means to an end, and I might almost say it is only weakening when it is made an end in itself.

Girls need to react intelligently to what is given them in physical training as much as to what is given them in a lecture on literature or philosophy or botany. How many girls do we know who take physical culture in a class, often simply because it is popular at the time, and never think of taking a long walk in the country—never think of going in for a vigorous outdoor game? How many girls do we know who take physical culture and never think of making life easy for their stomachs, or seeing that they get a normal amount of sleep? Exercise in the fresh air, with a hearty objective interest in all that is going on about us, is the very best sort of exercise that we can take, and physical culture is worse than nothing if it is not taken only as a means to enable us to do more in the open air, and do it better, and gain from it more life.

There is one girl who comes to my mind of whom I should like to tell because she illustrates truly a point that we cannot consider too carefully. She went to a nerve specialist very much broken in health, and when asked if she took plenty of exercise in the open air she replied "Yes, indeed." And it was proved to be the very best exercise. She had a good horse, and she rode well; she rode a great deal, and not too much. She had interesting dogs and she took them with her. She walked, too, in beautiful country. But she was carrying in her mind all the time extreme resistance to other circumstances of her life. She did not know how to drop the resistance or face the circumstances, and the mental strain in which she held herself day and night, waking or sleeping, prevented the outdoor exercise from really refreshing her. When she learned to face the circumstances then the exercise could do its good work.

On the other hand, there are many forms of nervous resistance and many disagreeable moods which good, vigorous exercise will blow away entirely, leaving our minds so clear that we wonder at ourselves, and wonder that we could ever have had those morbid thoughts.

The mind acts and the body reacts, the body acts and the mind reacts, but of course at the root of it all is the real desire for what is normal, or—alas!—the lack of that desire.

If physical culture does not make us love the open air, if it does not make us love to take a walk or climb a mountain, if it does not help us to take the walk or climb the mountain with more freedom, if it does not make us move along outdoors so easily that we forget our bodies altogether, and only enjoy what we see about us and feel how good it is to be alive—why, then physical culture is only an ornament without any use.

There is an interesting point in mountain-climbing which I should like to speak of, by the way, and which makes it much pleasanter and better exercise. If, after first starting—and, of course, you should start very slowly and heavily, like an elephant—you get out of breath, let yourself stay out of breath. Even emphasize the being out of breath by breathing harder than your lungs started to breathe, and then let your lungs pump and pump and pump until they find their own equilibrium. The result is delightful, and the physical freedom that follows is more than delightful. I remember seeing two girls climbing in the high Rocky Mountains in this way, when other women were going up on ponies. Finally one of the guides looked back, and with an expression of mild astonishment said "Well, you have lungs!" This was a very pleasant proof of the right kind of breathing.

There are many good points for climbing and walking and swimming and all outdoor exercise that can be gained from the best sort of physical culture; and physical culture is good for girls when it gives these points and leads to a spontaneous love for outdoor exercise. But when it results only in a self-conscious pose of the body then it is harmful.

We want to have strong bodies, free for every normal action, with quiet nerves, and muscles well coordinated. Then our bodies are merely instruments: good, clean, healthy instruments. They are the "mechanism of the outside." And when the mechanism of the outside is well oiled and running smoothly it can be forgotten.

There can be no doubt but that physical culture is good for girls provided it is given and taken with intelligent interest, but it must be done thoroughly to be done to real advantage. As, for instance, the part the shower-bath plays after exercising is most important, for it equalizes the circulation. Physical culture is good for girls who have little or no muscular action in their daily lives, for it gives them the healthiest exercise in the least space of time, and prepares them to get more life from exercise outdoors. It is good for girls whose daily lives are full of activity, because it develops the unused muscles and so rests those that have been overused. Many a hardworking girl has entered the gymnasium class tired and has left it rested.

CHAPTER XI

Working Restfully

ONCE met a man who had to do an important piece of scientific work in a given time. He worked from Saturday afternoon at 2 o'clock until Monday morning at 10 o'clock without interruption, except for one hour's sleep and the necessary time it took for nourishment.

After he had finished he was, of course, intensely tired, but instead of going right to bed and to sleep, and taking all that brain strain to sleep with him he took his dog and his gun and went hunting for several hours.

Turning his attention to something so entirely different gave the other part of his brain a chance to recover itself a little. The fresh air revived him, and the gentle exercise started up his circulation, If he had gone directly to sleep after his work, the chances are that it would have taken him days to recover from the fatigue, for nature would have had too much against her to have reacted quickly from so abnormal a strain—getting an entire change of attention and starting up his circulation in the fresh air gave nature just the start she needed. After that she could work steadily while he slept, and he awakened rested and refreshed.

To write from Saturday afternoon until Monday morning seems a stupid thing to do—no matter what the pressure is. To work for an abnormal time or at an abnormal rate is almost always stupid and short sighted.

There are exceptions, however, and it would be good if for those exceptions people knew how to take the best care of themselves. But it is not only after such abnormal work that we need to know how to react most restfully. It is important after all work, and especially for those who have some steady labor for the whole day.

Every one is more or less tired at the end of the day and the temptation is to drop into a chair or lie down on the sofa or to go right to bed and go to sleep. Don't do it.

Get some entire, active change for your brain, if it is only for fifteen minutes or half an hour. If you live in the city, even to go to walk and look into the shop windows is better than nothing. In that way you get fresh air, and if one knows how to look into shop windows without wanting anything or everything they see there, then it is very entertaining.

It is a good game to look into a shop window for two or three minutes and then look away and see how well you can remember everything in it. It is important always to take shop windows that are out of one's own line of work.

If you live in the country, a little walk out of doors is pleasanter than in the city, for the air is better; and there is much that is interesting, in the way of trees and sky, and stars, at night.

As you walk, make a conscious effort to look out and about you. Forget the work of the day, and take good long breaths.

When you do not feel like going out of doors, take a story book—or some other reading, if you prefer—and put your mind right on it for half an hour. The use of a really good novel cannot be overestimated. It not only serves as recreation, but it introduces us to phases of human nature that otherwise we would know nothing whatever about. A very great change from the day's work can be found in a good novel and a very happy change.

If the air in the theaters were fresher and good seats did not cost so much a good play, well acted, would be better than a good novel. Sometimes it freshens us up to play a game after the day's work is over, and for those who love music there is of course the greatest rest in that. But there again comes in the question of cost.

Why does not some kind soul start concerts for the people where, for a nominal admission, the best music can be heard? And why does not some other kind soul start a theater for the people where, for a very small price of admission, they can see the best plays and see them well acted?

We have public libraries in all our cities and towns, and a librarian in one large city loves to tell the tale of a poor woman in the slums with her door barred with furniture for fear of the drunken raiders in the house, quietly reading a book from the public library.

There are many similar stories to go with that. If we had really good theaters and really good concerts to be reached as simply and as easily as the books in our public libraries, the healthy influence throughout the cities would be proportionately increased. The trouble is that people cater as much to the rich with their ideas of a national theater as the theatrical syndicate itself.

I could not pretend to suggest amusements that would appeal to any or every reader, but I can make my point clear that when one is tired it is healthy to have a change of activity before going to rest.

"Oh," I hear, "I can't! I can't! I am too tired."

I know the feeling.

I have no doubt the man who wrote for nearly two days had a very strong tendency to go right to bed, but he had common sense behind it, and he knew the result would be better if he followed his common sense rather than his inclination. And so it proved.

It seems very hard to realize that it is not the best thing to go right to bed or to sit and do nothing when one is so tired as to make it seem impossible to do anything else.

It would be wrong to take vigorous physical exercise after great brain or body fatigue, but entire change of attention and gentle exercise is just what is needed, although care should always be taken not to keep at it too long. Any readers who make up their minds to try this process of resting will soon prove its happy effect.

A quotation from a recent daily paper reads, "'Rest while you work,' says Annie Payson Call,"—and then the editor adds, "and get fired," and although the opportunity for the joke was probably thought too good to lose, it was a natural misinterpretation of a very practical truth.

I can easily imagine a woman—especially a tired out and bitter woman—reading directions telling how to work restfully and exclaiming with all the vehemence of her bitterness: "That is all very well to write about. It sounds well, but let any one take hold of my work and try to do it restfully.

"If my employer should come along and see me working in a lazy way like that, he would very soon discharge me. No, no. I am tired out; I must keep at it as long as I can, and when I cannot keep at it any longer, I will die—and there is the end."

"It is nothing but drudge, drudge for your bread and butter—and what does your bread and butter amount to when you get it?"

There are thousands of women working to-day with bodies and minds so steeped in their fatigue that they cannot or will not take an idea outside of their rut of work. The rut has grown so deep, and they have sunken in so far that they cannot look over the edge.

It is true that it is easier to do good hard work in the lines to which one has been accustomed than to do easy work which is strange. Nerves will go on in old accustomed habits—even habits of tiresome strain—more easily than they will be changed into new habits of working without strain.

The mind, too, gets saturated with a sense of fatigue until the fatigue seems normal, and to feel well rested would—at first—seem abnormal. This being a fact, it is a logical result that an habitually tired and strained mind will indignantly refuse the idea that it can do more work and do it better without the strain.

There is a sharp corner to be turned to learn to work without strain, when one has had the habit of working with it. After the corner is turned, it requires steady, careful study to understand the new normal habit of working restfully, and to get the new habit established.

When once it is established, this normal habit of work develops its own requirements, and the working without strain becomes to us an essential part of the work itself.

For taken as a whole, more work is done and the work is done better when we avoid strain than when we do not. What is required to find this out is common sense and strength of character.

Character grows with practice; it builds and builds on itself when once it has a fair start, and a very little intelligence is needed if once the will is used to direct the body and mind in the lines of common sense.

Intelligence grows, too, as we use it. Everything good in the soul grows with use; everything bad, destroys.

Let us make a distinction to begin with between "rest while you work" and "working restfully."

"Rest while you work" might imply laziness. There is a time for rest and there is a time for work. When we work we should work entirely. When we rest we should rest entirely.

If we try to mix rest and work, we do neither well. That is true. But if we work restfully, we work then with the greatest amount of power and the least amount of effort.

That means more work and work better done after the right habit is established than we did before, when the wrong habit was established. The difficulty comes, and the danger of "getting fired," when we are changing our habit.

To obviate that difficulty, we must be content to change our habit more slowly. Suppose we come home Saturday night all tired out; go to bed and go to sleep, and wake Sunday almost more tired than when we went to bed. On Sunday we do not have to go to work.

Let us take a little time for the sole purpose of thinking our work over, and trying to find where the unnecessary strain is.

"But," I hear some one say, "I am too tired to think." Now it is a scientific fact that when our brains are all tired out in one direction, if we use our wills to start them working in another direction, they will get rested.

"But," again I hear, "if I think about my work, why isn't that using my brain in the same direction?" Because in thinking to apply new principles to work, of which you have never thought before, you are thinking in a new direction.

Not only that, but in applying new and true principles to your work you are bringing new life into the work itself.

On this Sunday morning, when you take an hour to devote yourself to the study of how you can work without getting overtired ask yourself the following questions:—

(1) "What do I resist in or about my work?" Find out each thing that you do resist, and drop the contractions that come in your body, with the intention of dropping the resistances in your mind.

(2) "Do I drop my work at meals and eat quietly?"

(3) "Do I take every opportunity that I can to get fresh air, and take good, full breaths of it?"

(4) "Do I feel hurried and pushed in my work? Do I realize that no matter how much of a hurry there may be, I can hurry more effectively if I drop the strain of the hurry?"

(5) "How much superfluous strain do I use in my work? Do I work with a feeling of strain? How can I observe better in order to become conscious of the strain and drop it?"

These are enough questions for one time! If you concentrate on these questions and on finding the answers, and do it diligently, you will be surprised to see how the true answers will come to you, and how much clearer they will become as you put them into daily practice.

CHAPTER XII

Imaginary Vacations

ONCE a young woman who had very hard work to do day after day and who had come to where she was chronically strained and tired, turned to her mother just as she was starting for work in the morning, and in a voice tense with fatigue and trouble, said:—

"Mother, I cannot stand it. I cannot stand it. Unless I can get a vacation long enough at least to catch my breath, I shall break down altogether."

"Why don't you take a vacation today?" asked her mother. The daughter got a little irritated and snapped out:—

"Why do you say such a foolish thing as that, Mother? You know as well as I that I could not leave my work today."

"Don't be cross, dear. Stop a minute and let me tell you what I mean. I have been thinking about it and I know you will appreciate what I have to say, and I know you can do it. Now listen." Whereupon the mother went on to explain quite graphically a process of pretense—good, wholesome pretense.

To any one who has no imagination this would not or could not appeal.

To the young woman of whom I write it not only appealed heartily, but she tried it and made it work. It was simply that she should play that she had commenced her vacation and was going to school to amuse herself.

As, for instance, she would say to herself, and believe it: "Isn't it good that I can have a vacation and a rest. What shall I do to get all I can out of it?

"I think I will go and see what they are doing in the grammar school. Maybe when I get there it will amuse me to teach some of the children. It is always interesting to see how children are going to take what you say to them and to see the different ways in which they recite their lessons."

By the time she got to school she was very much cheered. Looking up she said to herself: "This must be the building."

She had been in it every school day for five years past, but through the process of her little game it looked quite new and strange now.

She went in the door and when the children said "good morning," and some of them seemed glad to see her, she said to herself: "Why, they seem to know me; I wonder how that happens?" Occasionally she was so much amused at her own consistency in keeping up the game that she nearly laughed outright. She heard each class recite as if she were teaching for the first time. She looked upon each separate child as if she had never seen him before and he was interesting to her as a novel study.

She found the schoolroom more cheerful and was surprised into perceiving a pleasant sort of silent communication that started up between her pupils and herself.

When school was over she put on her hat and coat to go home, with the sense of having done something restful; and when she appeared to her mother, it was with a smiling, cheerful face, which made her mother laugh outright; and then they both laughed and went out for a walk in the fresh air, before coming in to go to bed, and be ready to begin again the next day.

In the morning the mother felt a little anxious and asked timidly: "Do you believe you can make it work again today, just as well as yesterday?"

"Yes, indeed and better," said the daughter. "It is too much fun not to go on with it."

After breakfast the mother with a little roguish twinkle, said: "Well, what do you think you will do to amuse yourself to-day, Alice?"

"Oh! I think—" and then they both laughed and Alice started off on her second day's "vacation."

By the end of a week she was out of that tired rut and having a very good time. New ideas had come to her about the school and the children; in fact, from being dead and heavy in her work, she had become alive.

When she found the old tired state coming on her again, she and her mother always "took a vacation," and every time avoided the tired rut more easily.

If one only has imagination enough, the helpfulness and restfulness of playing "take a vacation" will tell equally well in any kind of work.

You can play at dressmaking—play at millinery—play at keeping shop. You can make a game of any sort of drudgery, and do the work better for it, as well as keep better rested and more healthy yourself. But you must be steady and persistent and childlike in the way you play your game.

Do not stop in the middle and exclaim, "How silly!"—and then slump into the tired state again.

What I am telling you is nothing more nor less than a good healthy process of self-hypnotism. Really, it is more the attitude we take toward our work that tires us than the work itself. If we could only learn that and realize it as a practical fact, it would save a great deal of unnecessary suffering and even illness.

We do not need to play vacation all the time, of course. The game might get stale then and lose its power. If we play it for two or three days, whenever we get so tired that it seems as if we could not bear it—play it just long enough to lift ourselves out of the rut—then we can "go to work again" until we need another vacation.

We need not be afraid nor ashamed to bring back that childlike tendency—it will be of very great use to our mature minds.

If we try to play the vacation game, it is wiser to say nothing about it. It is not a game that we can be sure of sharing profitably either to ourselves or to others.

If you find it works, and give the secret to a friend, tell her to play it without mentioning it to you, even though she shares your work and is sitting in the next chair to you.

Another most healthy process of resting while you work is by means of lowering the pressure.

Suppose you were an engine, whose normal pressure was six hundred pounds, we will say. Make yourself work at a pressure of only three hundred pounds.

The human engine works with so much more strain than is necessary that if a woman gets overtired and tries to lighten her work by lightening the pressure with which she does it, she will find that really she has only thrown off the unnecessary strain, and is not only getting over her fatigue by working restfully, but is doing her work better, too.

In the process of learning to use less pressure, the work may seem to be going a little more slowly at first, but we shall find that it will soon go faster, and better, as time establishes the better habit.

One thing seems singular; and yet it appeals entirely to our common sense as we think of it. There never comes a time when we cannot learn to work more effectively at a lower pressure. We never get to where we cannot lessen our pressure and thus increase our power.

The very interest of using less pressure adds zest to our work, however it may have seemed like drudging before, and the possibility of resting while we work opens to us much that is new and refreshing, and gives us clearer understanding of how to rest more completely while we rest.

All kinds of resting, and all kinds of working, can bring more vitality than most of us know, until we have learned to rest and to work without strain.

CHAPTER XIII

The Woman at the Next Desk

IT may be the woman sewing in the next chair; it may be the woman standing next at the same counter; it may be the woman next at a working table, or it may be the woman at the next desk.

Whichever one it is, many a working woman has her life made wretched by her, and it would be a strange thing for this miserable woman to hear and a stranger thing—at first—for her to believe that the woman at the next desk need not trouble her at all.

That, if she only could realize it, the cause of the irritation which annoyed her every day and dragged her down so that many and many a night she had been home with a sick headache was entirely and solely in herself and not at all in the woman who worked next to her, however disagreeable that woman may have been.

Every morning when she wakes the woman at the next desk rises before her like a black specter. "Oh, I would not mind the work; I could work all day happily and quietly and go home at night and rest; the work would be a joy to me compared to this torture of having to live all day next to that woman."

It is odd, too, and true, that if the woman at the next desk finds that she is annoying our friend, unconsciously she seems to ferret out her most sensitive places and rub them raw with her sharp, discourteous words.

She seems to shirk her own work purposely and to arrange it so that the woman next her must do the work in her place. Then, having done all in her power to give the woman next her harder labor, she snaps out a little scornful remark about the mistakes that have been made.

If she—the woman at the next desk—comes in in the morning feeling tired and irritable herself, she vents her irritability on her companion until she has worked it off and goes home at night feeling much better herself, while her poor neighbor goes home tired out and weak.

The woman at the next desk takes pains to let little disagreeable hints drop about others—if not directly in their hearing at least in ways which she knows may reach them.

She drops hint to others of what those in higher office have said or appeared to think, which might frighten "others" quite out of their wits for fear of their being discharged, and then, where should they get their bread and butter?

All this and more that is frightful and disagreeable and mean may the woman at the next desk do; or she may be just plain, every-day *ugly*.

Every one knows the trying phases of her own working neighbor. But with all this, and with worse possibilities of harassment than I have even touched upon, the woman at the next desk is powerless, so far as I am concerned, if I choose to make her so.

The reason she troubles me is because I resist her. If she hurts my feelings, that is the same thing. I resist her, and the resistance, instead of making me angry, makes me sore in my nerves and makes me want to cry. The way to get independent of her is not to resist her, and the way to learn not to resist her is to make a daily and hourly study of dropping all resistances to her.

This study has another advantage, too; if we once get well started on it, it becomes so interesting that the concentration on this new interest brings new life in itself.

Resistance in the mind brings contraction in the body. If, when we find our minds resisting that which is disagreeable in another, we give our attention at once to finding the resultant contraction in our bodies, and then concentrate our wills on loosening out of the contraction, we cannot help getting an immediate result.

Even though it is a small result at the beginning, if we persist, results will grow until we, literally, find ourselves free from the woman at the next desk.

This woman says a disagreeable thing; we contract to it mind and body. We drop the contraction from our bodies, with the desire to drop it from our minds, for loosening the physical tension reacts upon the mental strain and relieves it.

We can say to ourselves quite cheerfully: "I wish she would go ahead and say another disagreeable thing; I should like to try the experiment again." She gives you an early opportunity and you try the experiment again, and again, and then again, until finally your brain gets the habit of trying the experiment without any voluntary effort on your part.

That habit being established, *you are free from the woman at the next desk.* She cannot irritate you nor wear upon you, no matter how she tries, no matter what she says, or what she does.

There is, however, this trouble about dropping the contraction. We are apt to have a feeling of what we might call "righteous indignation" at annoyances which are put upon us for no reason; that, so-called, "righteous indignation" takes the form of resistance and makes physical contractions.

It is useless to drop the physical contraction if the indignation is going to rise and tighten us all up again. If we drop the physical and mental contractions we must have something good to fill the open channels that have been made. Therefore let us give our best attention to our work, and if opportunity offers, do a kindness to the woman at the next desk.

Finally, when she finds that her ways do not annoy, she will stop them. She will probably, for a time at first, try harder to be disagreeable, and then after recovering from several surprises at not being able to annoy, she will quiet down and grow less disagreeable.

If we realize the effect of successive and continued resistance upon ourselves and realize at the same time that we can drop or hold those resistances as we choose to work to get free from them, or suffer and hold them, then we can appreciate the truth that if the woman at the next desk continues to annoy us, it is our fault entirely, and not hers.

CHAPTER XIV

Telephones and Telephoning

MOST men—and women—use more nervous force in speaking through the telephone than would be needed to keep them strong and healthy for years.

It is good to note that the more we keep in harmony with natural laws the more quiet we are forced to be.

Nature knows no strain. True science knows no strain. Therefore *a strained high-pitched voice does not carry over the telephone wire as well as a low one.*

If every woman using the telephone would remember this fact the good accomplished would be thricefold. She would save her own nervous energy. She would save the ears of the woman at the other end of the wire. She would make herself heard.

Patience, gentleness, firmness—a quiet concentration—all tell immeasurably over the telephone wire.

Impatience, rudeness, indecision, and diffuseness blur communication by telephone even more than they do when one is face to face with the person talking.

It is as if the wire itself resented these inhuman phases of humanity and spit back at the person who insulted it by trying to transmit over it such unintelligent bosh.

There are people who feel that if they do not get an immediate answer at the telephone they have a right to demand and get good service by means of an angry telephonic sputter.

The result of this attempt to scold the telephone girl is often an impulsive, angry response on her part—which she may be sorry for later on—and if the service is more prompt for that time it reacts later to what appears to be the same deficiency.

No one was ever kept steadily up to time by angry scolding. It is against reason.

To a demanding woman who is strained and tired herself, a wait of ten seconds seems ten minutes. I have heard such a woman ring the telephone bell almost without ceasing for fifteen minutes. I could hear her strain and anger reflected in the ringing of the bell. When finally she "got her party" the strain in her high-pitched voice made it impossible for her to be clearly understood. Then she got angry again because "Central" had not "given her a better connection," and finally came away from the telephone nearly in a state of nervous collapse and insisted that the telephone would finally end her life. I do not think she once suspected that the whole state of fatigue which had almost brought an illness upon her was absolutely and entirely her own fault.

The telephone has no more to do with it than the floor has to do with a child's falling and bumping his head.

The worst of this story is that if any one had told this woman that her tired state was all unnecessary, it would have roused more strain and anger, more fatigue, and more consequent illness.

Women must begin to find out their own deficiencies before they are ready to accept suggestions which can lead to greater freedom and more common sense.

Another place where science and inhuman humanity do not blend is in the angry moving up and down of the telephone hook.

When the hook is moved quickly and without pause it does not give time for the light before the telephone girl to flash, therefore she cannot be reminded that any one is waiting at the other end.

When the hook is removed with even regularity and a quiet pause between each motion then she can see the light and accelerate her action in getting "the other party."

I have seen a man get so impatient at not having an immediate answer that he rattled the hook up and down so fast and so vehemently as to nearly break it. There is something tremendously funny about this. The man is in a great hurry to speak to some one at the other end of the telephone, and yet he takes every means to prevent the operator from knowing what he wants by rattling his hook. In addition to this his angry movement of the hook is fast tending to break the telephone, so that he cannot use it at all. So do we interfere with gaining what we need by wanting it overmuch!

I do not know that there has yet been formed a telephone etiquette; but for the use of those who are not well bred by habit it would be useful to put such laws on the first page of the telephone book. A lack of consideration for others is often too evident in telephonic communication.

A woman will ask her maid to get the number of a friend's house for her and ask the friend to come to the telephone, and then keep her friend waiting while she has time to be called by the maid and to come to the telephone herself. This method of wasting other people's time is not confined to women alone. Men are equal offenders, and often greater ones, for the man at the other end is apt to be more immediately busy than a woman under such circumstances.

To sum up: The telephone may be the means of increasing our consideration for others; our quiet, decisive way of getting good service; our patience, and, through the low voice placed close to the transmitter, it may relieve us from nervous strain; for nerves always relax with the voice.

Or the telephone may be the means of making us more selfish and self-centered, more undecided and diffuse, more impatient, more strained and nervous.

In fact, the telephones may help us toward health or illness. We might even say the telephone may lead us toward heaven or toward hell. We have our choice of roads in the way we use it.

It is a blessed convenience and if it proves a curse—we bring the curse upon our own heads.

I speak of course only of the public who use the telephone. Those who serve the public in the use of the telephone must have many trials to meet, and, I dare say, are not always courteous and patient. But certainly there can be no case of lagging or discourtesy on the part of a telephone operator that is not promptly rectified by a quiet, decided appeal to the "desk."

It is invariably the nervous strain and the anger that makes the trouble.

There may be one of these days a school for the better use of the telephone; but such a school never need be established if every intelligent man and woman will be his and her own school in appreciating and acting upon the power gained if they compel themselves to go with science—and never allow themselves to go against it.

CHAPTER XV

Don't Talk

THERE is more nervous energy wasted, more nervous strain generated, more real physical harm done by superfluous talking than any one knows, or than any one could possibly believe who had not studied it. I am not considering the harm done by what people say. We all know the disastrous effects that follow a careless or malicious use of the tongue. That is another question. I simply write of the physical power used up and wasted by mere superfluous words, by using one hundred words where ten will do—or one thousand words where none at all were needed.

I once had been listening to a friend chatter, chatter, chatter to no end for an hour or more, when the idea occurred to me to tell her of an experiment I had tried by which my voice came more easily. When I could get an opportunity to speak, I asked her if she had ever tried taking a long breath and speaking as she let the breath out. I had to insist a little to keep her mind on the suggestion at all, but finally succeeded. She took a long breath and then stopped.

There was perhaps for half a minute a blessed silence, and then what was my surprise to hear her remark: "I—I—can't think of anything to say." "Try it again," I told her. She took another long breath, and again gave up because she could not think of anything to say. She did not like that little game very much, and thought she would not make another effort, and in about three minutes she began the chatter, and went on talking until some necessary interruption parted us.

This woman's talking was nothing more nor less than a nervous habit. Her thought and her words were not practically connected at all. She never said what she thought for she never thought. She never said anything in answer to what was said to her, for she never listened.

Nervous talkers never do listen. That is one of their most striking characteristics.

I knew of two well-known men—both great talkers—who were invited to dine. Their host thought, as each man talked a great deal and—, as he thought—talked very well, if they could meet their interchange of ideas would be most delightful. Several days later he met one of his guests in the street and asked how he liked the friend whom he had met for the first time at his house.

"Very pleasant, very pleasant," the man said, "but he talks too much."

Not long after this the other guest accosted him unexpectedly in the street "For Heaven's sake, don't ask me to dine with that Smith again—why, I could not get a word in edgewise."

Now, if only for selfish reasons a man might realize that he needs to absorb as well as give out, and so could make himself listen in order to be sure that his neighbor did not get ahead of him. But a conceited man, a self-centered man or a great talker will seldom or never listen.

That being the case, what can you expect of a woman who is a nervous talker? The more tired such a woman is the more she talks; the more ill she is the more she talks. As the habit of nervous talking grows upon a woman it weakens her mind. Indeed, nervous talking is a steadily weakening process.

Some women talk to forget. If they only knew it was slow mental suicide and led to worse than death they would be quick to avoid such false protection. If we have anything we want to forget we can only forget it by facing it until we have solved the problem that it places before us, and then working on, according to our best light: We can never really cover a thing up in our minds by talking constantly about something else.

Many women think they are going to persuade you of their point of view by talking. A woman comes to you with her head full of an idea and finds you do not agree with her. She will talk, talk, talk until you are blind and sick and heartily wish you were deaf, in order to prove to you that she is right and you are wrong.

She talks until you do not care whether you are right or wrong. You only care for the blessed relief of silence, and when she has left you, she has done all she could in that space of time to injure her point of view. She has simply buried anything good that she might have had to say in a cloud of dusty talk.

It is funny to hear such a woman say after a long interview, "Well, at any rate, I gave him a good talking to. I guess he will go home and think about it."

Think about it, madam? He will go home with an impression of rattle and chatter and push that will make him dread the sight of your face; and still more dread the sound of your voice, lest he be subjected to further interviews. Women sit at work together. One woman talks, talks, talks until her companions are so worn with the constant chatter that they have neither head nor nerve enough to do their work well. If they know how to let the chatter go on and turn their attention away from it, so that it makes no impression, they are fortunate indeed, and the practice is most useful to them. But that does not relieve the strain of the nervous talker herself; she is wearing herself out from day to day, and ruining her mind as well as hurting the nerves and dispositions of those about her who do not know how to protect themselves from her nervous talk.

Nervous talking is a disease.

Now the question is how to cure it. It can be cured, but the first necessity is for a woman to know she has the disease. For, unlike other diseases, the cure does not need a physician, but must be made by the patient herself.

First, she must know that she has the disease. Fifty nervous talkers might read this article, and not one of them recognize that it is aimed straight at her.

The only remedy for that is for every woman who reads to believe that she is a nervous talker until she has watched herself for a month or more—without prejudice—and has discovered for a certainty that she is not.

Then she is safe.

But what if she discover to her surprise and chagrin that she is a nervous talker? What is the remedy for that? The first thing to do is to own up the truth to herself without equivocation. To make no excuses or explanations but simply to acknowledge the fact.

Then let her aim straight at the remedy—silence—steady, severe, relaxed silence. Work from day to day and promise herself that for that day she will say nothing but what is absolutely necessary. She should not repress the words that want to come, but when she takes breath to speak she must not allow the sentence to come out of her mouth, but must instead relax all over, as far as it is possible, and take a good, long, quiet breath. The next time she wants to speak, even if she forgets so far as to get half the sentence out of her mouth, stop it, relax, and take a long breath.

The mental concentration necessary to cure one's self of nervous talking will gather together a mind that was gradually becoming dissipated with the nervous talking habit, and so the life and strength of the mind can be saved.

And, after that habit has been cured, the habit of quiet thinking will begin, and what is said will be worth while.

CHAPTER XVI

"Why Fuss so Much About What I Eat?"

I KNOW a woman who insisted that it was impossible for her to eat strawberries because they did not agree with her. A friend told her that that was simply a habit of her mind. Once, at a time when her stomach was tired or not in good condition for some other reason, strawberries had not agreed with her, and from that time she had taken it for granted that she could not eat strawberries. When she was convinced by her friend that her belief that strawberries did not agree with her was merely in her own idea, and not actually true, she boldly ate a plate of strawberries. That night she woke with indigestion, and the next morning she said "You see, I told you they would not agree with me."

But her friend answered: "Why, of course you could not expect them to agree right away, could you? Now try eating them again to-day."

This little lady was intelligent enough to want the strawberries to agree with her and to be willing to do her part to adjust herself to them, so she tried again and ate them the next day; and now she can eat them every day right through the strawberry season and is all the better for it.

This is the fact that we want to understand thoroughly and to look out for. If we are impressed with the idea that any one food does not agree with us, whenever we think of that food we contract, and especially our stomachs contract. Now if our stomachs contract when a food that we believe to disagree with us is merely mentioned, of course they would contract all the more when we ate it. Naturally our digestive organs would be handicapped by the contraction which came from our attitude of mind and, of course, the food would appear not to agree with us.

Take, for instance, people who are born with peculiar prenatal impressions about their food. A woman whom I have in mind could not take milk nor cream nor butter nor anything with milk or cream or butter in it. She seemed really proud of her milk-and-cream antipathy. She would air it upon all occasions, when she could do so without being positively discourteous, and often she came very near the edge of discourtesy. I never saw her even appear to make an effort to overcome it, and it is perfectly true that a prenatal impression like that can be overcome as entirely, as can a personally acquired impression, although it may take a longer time and a more persistent effort.

This anti-milk-and-cream lady was at work every day over-emphasizing her milk-and-cream contractions; whereas if she had put the same force into dropping the milk-and-cream contraction she would have been using her will to great advantage, and would have helped herself in many other ways as well as in gaining the ability to take normally a very healthful food. We cannot hold one contraction without having its influence draw us into many others. We cannot give our attention to dropping one contraction without having the influence of that one effort expand us in many other ways. Watch people when they refuse food that is passed them at table; you can see whether they refuse and at the same time contract against the food, or whether they refuse with no contraction at all. I have seen an expression of mild loathing on some women's faces when food was passed which "did not agree with them," but they were quite unconscious that their expressions had betrayed them.

Now, it is another fact that the contraction of the stomach at one form of food will interfere with the good digestion of another form. When cauliflower has been passed to us and we contract against it how can we expect our stomachs to recover from that contraction in time to digest perfectly the next vegetable which is passed and which we may like very much? It may be said that we expand to the vegetable we like, and that immediately counteracts the former contraction to the vegetable which we do not like. That is true only to a certain extent, for the tendency to cauliflower contraction is there in the back of our brains influencing our stomachs all the time, until we have actually used our wills consciously to drop it.

Edwin Booth used to be troubled very much with indigestion; he suffered keenly from it. One day he went to dine with some intimate friends, and before the dinner began his hostess said with a very smiling face: "Now, Mr. Booth, I have been especially careful with this dinner not to have one thing that you cannot digest."

The host echoed her with a hearty "Yes, Mr. Booth, everything that will come to the table is good for your digestion."

The words made a very happy impression on Mr. Booth. First there was the kind, sympathetic friendliness of his hosts; and then the strong suggestion they had given him that their food would agree with him. Then there was very happy and interesting talk during the whole time that they were at table and afterward. Mr.. Booth ate a hearty dinner and, true to the words of his host and hostess, not one single thing disagreed with him. And yet at that dinner, although care had been taken to have it wholesome, there were served things that under other conditions would have disagreed.

While we should aim always to eat wholesome food, it is really not so much the food which makes the trouble as the attitude we take toward it and the way we test it.

All the contractions which are made by our fussing about food interfere with our circulation; the interference with our circulation makes us liable to take cold, and it is safe to say that more than half the colds that women have are caused principally by wrong eating. Somewhat akin to grandmother's looking for her spectacles when all the time they are pushed to the top of her head is the way women fuss about their eating and then wonder why it is that they cannot seem to stand drafts.

There is no doubt but that our food should be thoroughly masticated before it goes into our stomachs. There is no doubt but that the first process of digestion should be in our mouths. The relish which we get for our food by masticating it properly is greater and also helps toward digesting it truly. All this cannot be over-emphasized if it is taken in the right way. But there is an extreme which perhaps has not been thought of and for which happily I have an example that will illustrate what I want to prove. I know a woman who was, so to speak, daft on the subject of health. She attended to all points of health with such minute detail that she seemed to have lost all idea of why we should be healthy. One of her ways of over-emphasizing the road to health was a very careful mastication of her food. She chewed and chewed and chewed and chewed, and the result was that she so strained her stomach with her chewing that she brought on severe indigestion, simply as a result of an overactive effort toward digestion. This was certainly a case of "vaulting ambition, which o'erleaps itself, and falls on the other." And it was not unique.

The over-emphasis of "What shall I eat? How much shall I eat? How often shall I eat? When shall I eat? How shall I eat?"—all extreme attention to these questions is just as liable to bring chronic indigestion as a reckless neglect of them altogether is liable to upset a good, strong stomach and keep it upset. The woman who chewed herself into indigestion fussed herself into it, too, by constantly talking about what was not healthful to eat. Her breakfast, which she took alone, was for a time the dryest-looking meal I ever saw. It was enough to take away any one's healthy relish just to look at it, if he was not forewarned.

Now our relish is one of our most blessed gifts. When we relish our food our stomachs can digest it wholesomely. When we do not our stomachs will not produce the secretions necessary to the most wholesome digestion. Constant fussing about our food takes away our relish. A gluttonous dwelling upon our food takes away our relish. Relish is a delicate gift, and as we respect it truly, as we do not degrade it to selfish ends nor kill it with selfish fastidiousness, it grows upon us and is in its place like any other fine perception, and is as greatly useful to the health of our bodies as our keener and deeper perceptions are useful to the health of our minds.

Then there is the question of being sure that our stomachs are well rested before we give them any work to do, and being sure that we are quiet enough after eating to give our stomachs the best opportunity to begin their work. Here again one extreme is just as harmful as the other. I knew a woman who had what might be called the fixed idea of health, who always used to sit bolt upright in a high-backed chair for half an hour after dinner, and refuse to speak or to be spoken to in order that "digestion might start in properly." If I had been her stomach I should have said: "Madam, when you have got through giving me your especial attention I will begin my work—which, by the way, is not your work but mine!" And, virtually, that is what her stomach did say. Sitting bolt upright and consciously waiting for your food to begin digestion is an over-attention to what is none of your business, which contracts your brain, contracts your stomach and stops its work.

Our business is only to fulfill the conditions rightly. The French workmen do that when they sit quietly after a meal talking of their various interests. Any one can fulfill the conditions properly by keeping a little quiet, having some pleasant chat, reading a bright story or taking life easy in any quiet way for half an hour. Or, if work must begin directly after eating, begin it quietly. But this feeling that it is our business to attend to the working functions of our stomachs is officious and harmful. We must fulfill the conditions and then forget our stomachs. If our stomachs remind us of themselves by some misbehavior we must seek for the cause and remedy it, but we should not on any account feel that the cause is necessarily in the food we have eaten. It may be, and probably often is, entirely back of that. A quick, sharp resistance to something that is said will often cause indigestion. In that case we must stop resisting and not blame the food. A dog was once made to swallow a little bullet with his food and then an X-ray was thrown on to his stomach in order that the process of digestion might be watched by means of the bullet. When the dog was made angry the bullet stopped, which meant that the digestion stopped; when the dog was over-excited in any way digestion stopped. When he was calmed down it went on again.

There are many reasons why we should learn to meet life without useless resistance, and the health of our stomachs is not the least.

It would surprise most people if they could know how much unnecessary strain they put on their stomachs by eating too much. A nervous invalid had a very large appetite. She was helped twice, sometimes three times, to meat and vegetables at dinner. She thought that what she deemed her very healthy appetite was a great blessing to her, and often remarked upon it, as also upon her idea that so much good, nourishing food must be helping to make her well. And yet she wondered why she did not gain faster.

Now the truth of the matter was that this invalid had a nervous appetite. Not only did she not need one third of the food she ate, but indeed the other two thirds was doing her positive harm. The tax which she put upon her stomach to digest so much food drained her nerves every day, and of course robbed her brain, so that she ate and ate and wept and wept with nervous depression. When it was suggested to her by a friend who understood nerves that she would get better very much faster if she would eat very much less she made a rule to take only one helping of anything, no matter how much she might feel that she wanted another. Very soon she began to gain enough to see for herself that she had been keeping herself ill with overeating, and it was not many days before she did not want a second helping.

Nervous appetites are not uncommon even among women who consider themselves pretty well. Probably there are not five in a hundred among all the well-fed men and women in this country who would not be more healthy if they ate less.

Then there are food notions to be looked out for and out of which any one can relax by giving a little intelligent attention to the task.

"I do not like eggs. I am tired of them." "Dear, dear me! I ate so much ice cream that it made me ill, and it has made me ill to think of it ever since."

Relax, drop the contraction, pretend you had never tasted ice cream before, and try to eat a little—not for the sake of the ice cream, but for the sake of getting that knot out of your stomach.

"But," you will say, "can every one eat everything?"

"Yes," the answer is, "everything that is really good, wholesome food is all right for anybody to eat."

But you say: "Won't you allow for difference of tastes?"

And the answer to that is: "Of course we can like some foods more than others, but there is a radical difference between unprejudiced preferences and prejudiced dislikes."

Our stomachs are all right if we will but fulfill their most simple conditions and then leave them alone. If we treat them right they will tell us what is good for them and what is not good for them, and if we will only pay attention, obey them as a matter of course without comment and then forget them, there need be no more fuss about food and very much less nervous irritability.

CHAPTER XVII

Take Care of Your Stomach

WE all know that we have a great deal to do. Some of us have to work all day to earn our bread and butter and then work a good part of the night to make our clothes. Some of us have to stand all day behind a counter. Some of us have to sit all day and sew for others, and all night to sew for ourselves and our children. Most of us have to do work that is necessary or work that is self-imposed. Many of us feel busy without really being busy at all. But how many of us realize that while we are doing work outside, our bodies themselves have good, steady work to do inside.

Our lungs have to take oxygen from the air and give it to our blood; our blood has to carry it all through our bodies and take away the waste by means of the steady pumping of our hearts. Our stomachs must digest the food put into them, give the nourishment in it to the blood, and see that the waste is cast off.

All this work is wholesome and good, and goes on steadily, giving us health and strength and new power; but if we, through mismanagement, make heart or lungs or stomach work harder than they should, then they must rob us of power to accomplish what we give them to do, and we blame them, instead of blaming ourselves for being hard and unjust taskmasters.

The strain in a stomach necessary to the digesting of too much food, or the wrong kind of food, makes itself felt in strain all through the whole system.

I knew a woman whose conscience was troubling her very greatly. She was sure she had done many very selfish things for which there was no excuse, and that she herself was greatly to blame for other people's troubles. This was a very acute attack of conscience, accompanied by a very severe stomach ache. The doctor was called in and gave her an emetic. She threw a large amount of undigested food from her stomach, and after that relief the weight on her conscience was lifted entirely and she had nothing more to blame herself with than any ordinary, wholesome woman must have to look out for every day of her life.

This is a true story and should be practically useful to readers who need it. This woman's stomach had been given too much to do. It worked hard to do its work well, and had to rob the brain and nervous system in the effort. This effort brought strain to the whole brain, which was made evident in the region of the conscience. It might have come out in some other form. It might have appeared in irritability. It might even have shown itself in downright ugliness.

Whatever the effects are, whether exaggerated conscience, exaggerated anxiety, or irritability, the immediate cause of the trouble in such cases as I refer to is in the fact that the stomach has been given too much to do.

We give the stomach too much to do if we put a great deal of food into it when it is tired. We give it too much to do if we put into it the wrong kind of food. We give it too much to do if we insist upon working hard ourselves, either with body or brain, directly after a hearty meal.

No matter how busy we are we can protect our stomachs against each and all of these three causes of trouble.

If a woman is very tired her stomach must necessarily be very tired also. If she can remember that at such times even though she may be very hungry, her body is better nourished if she takes slowly a cup of hot milk, and waits until she is more rested before taking solid food, than if she ate a hearty meal. It will save a strain, and perhaps eventually severe illness.

If it is possible to rest and do absolutely nothing for half an hour before a meal, and for half an hour after that insures the best work for our digestion. If one is pretty well, and cannot spare the half hour, ten or fifteen minutes will do, unless there is a great deal of fatigue to be conquered.

If it is necessary to work right up to mealtime, let up a little before stopping. As the time for dinner approaches do not work quite so hard; the work will not lose; in the end it will gain—and when you begin work again begin lightly, and get into the thick of it gradually. That gives your stomach a good chance.

If possible get a long rest before the last meal, and if your day is very busy, it is better to have the heartiest meal at the end of it, to take a good rest afterward and then a walk in the fresh air, which may be long or short, according to what other work you have to do or according to how tired you are.

I know many women will say: "But I am tired all the time; if I waited to rest before I ate, I should starve."

The answer to that is "protect your stomach as well as you can. If you cannot rest before and after each meal try to arrange some way by which you can get rid of a little fatigue."

If you do this with attention and interest you will find gradually that you are less tired all the time, and as you keep on steadily toward the right path, you may be surprised some day to discover that you are only tired half the time, and perhaps even reach the place where the tired feeling will be the exception.

It takes a good while to get our misused stomachs into wholesome ways, but if we are persistent and intelligent we can surely do it, and the relief to the overstrained stomach—as I have said—means relief to the whole body.

Resting before and after meals amounts to very little, however, if we eat food that is not nourishing.

Some people are so far out of the normal way of eating that they have lost a wholesome sense of what is good for them, and live in a chronic state of disordered stomach, which means a chronic state of disordered nerves and disposition. If such persons could for one minute literally experience the freedom of a woman whose body was truly and thoroughly nourished, the contrast from the abnormal to the normal would make them dizzy. If, however, they stayed in the normal place long enough to get over the dizziness, the freedom of health would be so great a delight that food that was not nourishing would be nauseous to them.

Most of us are near enough the normal to know the food that is best for us, through experience of suffering from food which is not best for us, as well as through good natural instinct.

If we would learn from the normal working of the involuntary action of our organs, it might help us greatly toward working more wholesomely in all our voluntary actions.

If every woman who reads this article would study not to interfere with the most healthy action of her own stomach, her reward after a few weeks' persistent care would be not only a greater power for work, but a greater power for good, healthy, recuperative rest.

CHAPTER XVIII

About Faces

WATCH the faces as you walk along the street! If you get the habit of noticing, your observations will grow keener. It is surprising to see how seldom we find a really quiet face. I do not mean that there should be no lines in the face. We are here in this world at school and we cannot have any real schooling unless we have real experiences. We cannot have real experiences without suffering, and suffering which comes from the discipline of life and results in character leaves lines in our faces. It is the lines made by unnecessary strain to which I refer.

Strange to say the unquiet faces come mostly from shallow feeling. Usually the deeper the feeling the less strain there is on the face. A face may look troubled, it may be full of pain, without a touch of that strain which comes from shallow worry or excitement.

The strained expression takes character out of the face, it weakens it, and certainly it detracts greatly from whatever natural beauty there may have been to begin with. The expression which comes from pain or any suffering well borne gives character to the face and adds to its real beauty as well as its strength.

To remove the strained expression we must remove the strain behind; therefore the hardest work we have to do is below the surface. The surface work is comparatively easy.

I know a woman whose face is quiet and placid. The lines are really beautiful, but they are always the same. This woman used to watch herself in the glass until she had her face as quiet and free from lines as she could get it—she used even to arrange the corners of her mouth with her fingers until they had just the right droop.

Then she observed carefully how her face felt with that placid expression and studied to keep it always with that feeling, until by and by her features were fixed and now the placid face is always there, for she has established in her brain an automatic vigilance over it that will not allow the muscles once to get "out of drawing."

What kind of an old woman this acquaintance of mine will make I do not know. I am curious to see her—but now she certainly is a most remarkable hypocrite. The strain in behind the mask of a face which she has made for herself must be something frightful. And indeed I believe it is, for she is ill most of the time—and what could keep one in nervous illness more entirely than this deep interior strain which is necessary to such external appearance of placidity.

There comes to my mind at once a very comical illustration of something quite akin to this although at first thought it seems almost the reverse. A woman who constantly talked of the preeminency of mind over matter, and the impossibility of being moved by external circumstances to any one who believed as she did—this woman I saw very angry.

She was sitting with her face drawn in a hundred cross lines and all askew with her anger. She had been spouting and sputtering what she called her righteous indignation for some minutes, when after a brief pause and with the angry expression still on her face she exclaimed: "Well, I don't care, it's all peace within."

I doubt if my masked lady would ever have declared to herself or to any one else that "it was all peace within." The angry woman was—without doubt—the deeper hypocrite, but the masked woman had become rigid in her hypocrisy. I do not know which was the weaker of the two, probably the one who was deceiving herself.

But to return to those drawn, strained lines we see on the people about us. They do not come from hard work or deep thought. They come from unnecessary contractions about the work. If we use our wills consistently and steadily to drop such contractions, the result is a more quiet and restful way of living, and so quieter and more attractive faces.

This unquietness comes especially in the eyes. It is a rare thing to see a really quiet eye; and very pleasant and beautiful it is when we do see it. And the more we see and observe the unquiet eyes and the unquiet faces the better worth while it seems to work to have ours more quiet, but not to put on a mask, or be in any other way a hypocrite.

The exercise described in a previous chapter will help to bring a quiet face. We must drop our heads with a sense of letting every strain go out of our faces, and then let our heads carry our bodies down as far as possible, dropping strain all the time, and while rising slowly we must take the same care to drop all strain.

In taking the long breath, we must inhale without effort, and exhale so easily that it seems as if the breath went out of itself, like the balloons that children blow up and then watch them shrink as the air leaves them.

Five minutes a day is very little time to spend to get a quiet face, but just that five minutes—if followed consistently—will make us so much more sensitive to the unquiet that we will sooner or later turn away from it as by a natural instinct.

CHAPTER XIX

About Voices

I KNEW an old German—a wonderful teacher of the speaking voice—who said "the ancients believed that the soul of the man is here"—pointing to the pit of his stomach. "I do not know," and he shrugged his shoulders with expressive interest, "it may be and it may not be—but I know the soul of the voice is here—and you Americans—you squeeze the life out of the word in your throat and it is born dead."

That old artist spoke the truth—we Americans—most of us—do squeeze the life out of our words and they are born dead. We squeeze the life out by the strain which runs all through us and reflects itself especially in our voices.

Our throats are tense and closed; our stomachs are tense and strained; with many of us the word is dead before it is born.

Watch people talking in a very noisy place; hear how they scream at the top of their lungs to get above the noise. Think of the amount of nervous force they use in their efforts to be heard.

Now really when we are in the midst of a great noise and want to be heard, what we have to do is to pitch our voices on a different key from the noise about us. We can be heard as well, and better, if we pitch our voices on a lower key than if we pitch them on a higher key; and to pitch your voice on a low key requires very much less effort than to strain to a high one.

I can imagine talking with some one for half an hour in a noisy factory—for instance—and being more rested at the end of the half hour than at the beginning. Because to pitch your voice low you must drop some superfluous tension and dropping superfluous tension is always restful.

I beg any or all of my readers to try this experiment the next time they have to talk with a friend in a noisy street. At first the habit of screaming above the noise of the wheels is strong on us and it seems impossible that we should be heard if we speak below it. It is difficult to pitch our voices low and keep them there. But if we persist until we have formed a new habit, the change is delightful.

There is one other difficulty in the way; whoever is listening to us may be in the habit of hearing a voice at high tension and so find it difficult at first to adjust his ear to the lower voice and will in consequence insist that the lower tone cannot be heard as easily.

It seems curious that our ears can be so much engaged in expecting screaming that they cannot without a positive effort of the mind readjust in order to listen to a lower tone. But it is so. And, therefore, we must remember that to be thoroughly successful in speaking intelligently below the noise we must beg our listeners to change the habit of their ears as we ourselves must change the pitch of our voices.

The result both to speaker and listener is worth the effort ten times over.

As we habitually lower the pitch of our voices our words cease gradually to be "born dead." With a low-pitched voice everything pertaining to the voice is more open and flexible and can react more immediately to whatever may be in our minds to express.

Moreover, the voice itself may react back again upon our dispositions. If a woman gets excited in an argument, especially if she loses her temper, her voice will be raised higher and higher until it reaches almost a shriek. And to hear two women "argue" sometimes it may be truly said that we are listening to a "caterwauling." That is the only word that will describe it.

But if one of these women is sensitive enough to know she is beginning to strain in her argument and will lower her voice and persist in keeping it lowered the effect upon herself and the other woman will put the "caterwauling" out of the question.

"Caterwauling" is an ugly word. It describes an ugly sound. If you have ever found yourself in the past aiding and abetting such an ugly sound in argument with another—say to yourself "caterwauling," "caterwauling," "I have been 'caterwauling' with Jane Smith, or Maria Jones," or whoever it may be, and that will bring out in such clear relief the ugliness of the word and the sound that you will turn earnestly toward a more quiet way of speaking.

The next time you start on the strain of an argument and your voice begins to go up, up, up—something will whisper in your ear "caterwauling" and you will at once, in self-defense, lower your voice or stop speaking altogether.

It is good to call ugly things by their ugliest names. It helps us to see them in their true light and makes us more earnest in our efforts to get away from them altogether.

I was once a guest at a large reception and the noise of talking seemed to be a roar, when suddenly an elderly man got up on a chair and called "silence," and having obtained silence he said, "it has been suggested that every one in this room should speak in a lower tone of voice."

The response was immediate. Every one went on talking with the same interest only in a lower tone of voice with a result that was both delightful and soothing.

I say every one—there were perhaps half a dozen whom I observed who looked and I have no doubt said "how impudent." So it was "impudent" if you chose to take it so—but most of the people did not choose to take it so and so brought a more quiet atmosphere and a happy change of tone.

Theophile Gautier said that the voice was nearer the soul than any other expressive part of us. It is certainly a very striking indicator of the state of the soul. If we accustom ourselves to listen to the voices of those about us we detect more and more clearly various qualities of the man or the woman in the voice, and if we grow sensitive to the strain in our own voices and drop it at once when it is perceived, we feel a proportionate gain.

I knew of a blind doctor who habitually told character by the tone of the voice, and men and women often went to him to have their characters described as one would go to a palmist.

Once a woman spoke to him earnestly for that purpose and he replied, "Madam, your voice has been so much cultivated that there is nothing of you in it—I cannot tell your real character at all." The only way to cultivate a voice is to open it to its best possibilities—not to teach its owner to pose or to imitate a beautiful tone until it has acquired the beautiful tone habit. Such tones are always artificial and the unreality in them can be easily detected by a quick ear.

Most great singers are arrant hypocrites. There is nothing of themselves in their tone. The trouble is to have a really beautiful voice one must have a really beautiful soul behind it.

If you drop the tension of your voice in an argument for the sake of getting a clearer mind and meeting your opponent without resistance, your voice helps your mind and your mind helps your voice.

They act and react upon one another with mutual benefit. If you lower your voice in general for the sake of being more quiet, and so more agreeable and useful to those about you, then again the mental or moral effort and the physical effort help one another.

It adds greatly to a woman's attraction and to her use to have a low, quiet voice—and if any reader is persisting in the effort to get five minutes absolute quiet in every day let her finish the exercise by saying something in a quiet, restful tone of voice.

It will make her more sensitive to her unrestful tones outside, and so help her to improve them.

CHAPTER XX

About Frights

HERE are two true stories and a remarkable contrast. A nerve specialist was called to see a young girl who had had nervous prostration for two years. The physician was told before seeing the patient that the illness had started through fright occasioned by the patient's waking and discovering a burglar in her room.

Almost the moment the doctor entered the sick room, he was accosted with: "Doctor, do you know what made me ill? It was frightful." Then followed a minute description of her sudden awakening and seeing the man at her bureau drawers.

This story had been lived over and over by the young girl and her friends for two years, until the strain in her brain caused by the repetition of the impression of fright was so intense that no skill nor tact seemed able to remove it. She simply would not let it go, and she never got really well.

Now, see the contrast. Another young woman had a similar burglar experience, and for several nights after she woke with a start at the same hour. For the first two or three nights she lay and shivered until she shivered herself to sleep.

Then she noticed how tightened up she was in every muscle when she woke, and she bethought herself that she would put her mind on relaxing her muscles and getting rid of the tension in her nerves. She did this persistently, so that when she woke with the burglar fright it was at once a reminder to relax.

After a little she got the impression that she woke in order to relax and it was only a very little while before she succeeded so well that she did not wake until it was time to get up in the morning.

The burglar impression not only left her entirely, but left her with the habit of dropping all contractions before she went to sleep, and her nerves are stronger and more normal in consequence.

The two girls had each a very sensitive, nervous temperament, and the contrast in their behavior was simply a matter of intelligence.

This same nerve specialist received a patient once who was positively blatant in her complaint of a nervous shock. "Doctor, I have had a horrible nervous shock. It was horrible. I do not see how I can ever get over it."

Then she told it and brought the horrors out in weird, over-vivid colors. It was horrible, but she was increasing the horrors by the way in which she dwelt on it.

Finally, when she paused long enough to give the doctor an opportunity to speak, he said, very quietly: "Madam, will you kindly say to me, as gently as you can, 'I have had a severe nervous shock.'" She looked at him without a gleam of understanding and repeated the words quietly: "I have had a severe nervous shock."

In spite of herself she felt the contrast in her own brain. The habitual blatancy was slightly checked. The doctor then tried to impress upon her the fact that she was constantly increasing the strain of the shock by the way she spoke of it and the way she thought of it, and that she was really keeping herself ill.

Gradually, as she learned to relax the nervous tension caused by the shock, a true intelligence about it all dawned upon her; the over-vivid colors faded, and she got well. She was surprised herself at the rapidity with which she got well, but she seemed to understand the process and to be moderately grateful for it.

If she had had a more sensitive temperament she would have appreciated it all the more keenly; but if she had had a more sensitive temperament she would not have been blatant about her shock.

CHAPTER XXI

Contrariness

I KNOW a woman who says that if she wants to get her father's consent to anything, she not only appears not to care whether he consents or not, but pretends that her wishes are exactly opposite to what they really are. She says it never fails; the decision has always been made in opposition to her expressed desires, and according to her real wishes. In other words, she has learned how to manage her father.

This example is not unique. Many of us see friends managing other friends in that same way. The only thing which can interfere with such astute management is the difficulty that a man may have in concealing his own will in order to accomplish what he desires. Wilfulness is such an impulsive quantity that it will rush ahead in spite of us and spoil everything when we feel that there is danger of our not getting our own way. Or, if we have succeeded in getting our own way by what might be called the "contrary method," we may be led into an expression of satisfaction which will throw light on the falseness of our previous attitude and destroy the confidence of the friend whom we were tactfully influencing.

To work the "contrary method" to perfection requires a careful control up to the finish and beyond it. In order never to be found out, we have to be so consistent in our behavior that we gradually get trained into nothing but a common every-day hypocrite, and the process which goes on behind hypocrisy must necessarily be a process of decay. Beside that, the keenest hypocrite that ever lived can only deceive others up to a certain limit.

But what is one to do when a friend can only be reached by the "contrary method"? What is one to do when if, for instance, you want a friend to read a book, you know that the way to prevent his reading it is to mention your desire? If you want a friend to see a play and in a forgetful mood mention the fact that you feel sure the play would delight him, you know as soon as the words are out of your mouth you have put the chance of his seeing the play entirely out of the question? What is one to do when something needs mending in the house, and you know that to mention the need to the man of the house would be to delay the repair just so much longer? How are our contrary-minded friends to be met if we cannot pretend we do not want what we do want in order to get their cooperation and consent?

No one could deliberately plan to be a hypocrite understanding what a hypocrite really is. A hypocrite is a sham—a sham has nothing solid to stand on. No one really respects a sham, and the most intelligent, the most tactful hypocrite that ever lived is nothing but a sham,—*false* and a sham!

Beside, no one can manage another by the process of sham and hypocrisy without sooner or later being found out, and when he is found out, all his power is gone.

The trouble with the contrary-minded is they have an established habit of resistance. Sometimes the habit is entirely inherited, and has never been seen or acknowledged. Sometimes it has an inherited foundation, with a cultivated superstructure.

Either way it is a problem for those who have to deal with it,—until they understand. The "contrary method" does not solve the problem; it is only a makeshift; it never does any real work, or accomplishes any real end. It is not even lastingly intelligent.

The first necessity in dealing truly with these people is *not to be afraid of their resistances*. The second necessity, which is so near the first that the two really belong side by side, is *never to meet their resistances with resistances of our own*.

If we combat another man's resistance, it only increases his tension. No matter how wrong he may be, and how right we are, meeting resistance with resistance only breeds trouble. Two minds can act and react upon one another in that way until they come to a lock which not only makes lasting enemies of those who should have been and could be always friends, but the contention locks up strain in each man's brain which can never be removed without pain, and a new awakening to the common sense of human intercourse.

If we want a friend to read a book, to go a journey, or to do something which is more important for his own good than either, and we know that to suggest our desire would be to rouse his resistance, the only way is to catch him in the best mood we can, say what we have to say, give our own preference, and at the same time feel and express a willingness to be refused. Every man is a free agent, and we have no right not to respect his freedom, even if he uses that freedom to stand in his own light or in ours. If he is standing in our light and refuses to move, we can move out of his shadow, even though we may have to give up our most cherished desire in order to do so.

If he is standing in his own light, and refuses to move, we can suggest or advise and do whatever in us lies to make the common sense of our opinion clear; but if he still persists in standing in his own light, it is his business, not ours.

It requires the cultivation of a strong will to put a request before a friend which we know will be resisted, and to yield to that resistance so that it meets no antagonism in us. But when it is done, and done thoroughly, consistently, and intelligently, the other man's resistance reacts back upon himself, and he finds himself out as he never could in any other way. Having found himself out, unless his mulishness is almost past sanity, he begins to reject his habit of resistance of his own accord.

In dealing with the contrary minded, the "contrary method" works so long as it is not discovered; and the danger of its being discovered is always imminent. The upright, direct method is according to the honorable laws of human intercourse, and brings always better results in the end, even though there may be some immediate failures in the process.

To adjust ourselves rightly to another nature and go with it to a good end, along the lines of least resistance, is of course the best means of a real acquaintance, but to allow ourselves to manage a fellow-being is an indignity to the man and worse than an indignity to the mind who is willing to do the managing.

Our humanity is in our freedom. Our freedom is in our humanity. When one, man tries to manage another, he is putting that other in the attitude of a beast. The man who is allowing himself to be managed is classing himself with the beasts.

Although this is a fact so evident on the base of it that it needs neither explanation nor enlargement, there is hardly a day passes that some one does not say to some one, "You cannot manage me in that way," and the answer should be, "Why should you want to be managed in any way; and why should I want to insult you by trying to manage you at all?"

The girl and her father might have been intelligent friends by this time, if the practice of the "contrary method" had not tainted the girl with habitual hypocrisy, and cultivated in the father the warped mind which results from the habit of resistance, and blind weakness which comes from the false idea that he is always having his own way.

If we want an open brain and a good, freely working nervous system, we must respect our own freedom and the freedom of other people,—for only as individuals stand alone can they really influence one another to any good end.

It is curious to see how the men of habitual resistance pride themselves on being in bondage to no one, not knowing that the fear of such bondage is what makes them resist, and the fear of being influenced by another is one of the most painful forms of bondage in which a man can be.

The men who are slaves to this fear do not stop even to consider the question. They resist and refuse a request at once, for fear that pausing for consideration would open them to the danger of appearing to yield to the will of another.

When we are quite as willing to yield to another as to refuse him, then we are free, and can give any question that is placed before us intelligent consideration, and decide according to our best judgment. No amount of willfulness can force a man to any action or attitude of mind if he is willing to yield to the willful pressure if it seems to him best.

The worse bondage of man to man is the bondage of fear.

CHAPTER XXII

How to Sew Easily

IT is a common saying that we should let our heads save our heels, but few of us know the depth of it or the freedom and health that can come from obedience to it.

For one thing we get into ruts. If a woman grows tired sewing she takes it for granted that she must always be tired. Sometimes she frets and complains, which only adds to her fatigue.

Sometimes she goes on living in a dogged state of overtiredness until there comes a "last straw" which brings on some organic disease, and still another "straw" which kills her altogether.

We, none of us, seem to realize that our heads can save not only our heels, but our hearts, and our lungs, our spines and our brains—indeed our whole nervous systems.

Men and women sometimes seem to prefer to go on working—chronically tired—getting no joy from life whatever, rather than to take the trouble to think enough to gain the habit of working restfully.

Sometimes, to be sure, they are so tired that the little extra exertion of the brain required to learn to get rid of the fatigue seems too much for them.

It seems easier to work in a rut of strain and discomfort than to make the effort to get out of the rut—even though they know that by doing so they will not only be better themselves, but will do their work better.

Now really the action of the brain which is needed to help one to work restfully is quite distinct from the action which does the work, and a little effort of the brain in a new direction rests and refreshes the part of the brain which is drudging along day after day, and not only that, but when one has gained the habit of working more easily life is happier and more worth while. If once we could become convinced of that fact it would be a simple matter for the head to learn to save the heels and for the whole body to be more vigorous in consequence.

Take sewing, for instance: If a woman must sew all day long without cessation and she can appreciate that ten or fifteen minutes taken out of the day once in the morning and once in the afternoon is going to save fatigue and help her to do her sewing better, doesn't it seem simply a lack of common sense if she is not willing to take that half hour and use it for its right purpose? Or, if she is employed with others, is it not a lack of common sense combined with cruelty in her employer if he will not permit the use of fifteen minutes twice a day to help his employees to do their work better and to keep more healthy in the process of working?

It seems to me that all most of us need is to have our attention drawn to the facts in such cases as this and then we shall be willing and anxious to correct the mistakes.

First, we do not know, and, secondly, we do not think, intelligently. It is within our reach to do both.

Let me put the facts about healthy sewing in numerical order:—

First—A woman should never sew nor be allowed to sew in bad air. The more or less cramped attitude of the chest in sewing makes it especially necessary that the lungs should be well supplied with oxygen, else the blood will lose vitality, the appetite will go and the nerves will be straining to bring the muscles up to work which they could do quite easily if they were receiving the right amount of nourishment from air and food.

Second—When our work gives our muscles a tendency steadily in one direction we must aim to counteract that tendency by using exercises with a will to pull them in the opposite way.

If a man writes constantly, to stop writing half a dozen times a day and stretch the fingers of his hand wide apart and let them relax back slowly will help him so that he need not be afraid of writer's paralysis.

Now a woman's tendency in sewing is to have her chest contracted and settled down on her stomach, and her head bent forward. Let her stop even twice a day, lift her chest off her stomach, see that the lifting of her chest takes her shoulders back, let her head gently fall back, take a long quiet breath in that attitude, then bring the head up slowly, take some long quiet breaths like gentle sighs, gradually let the lungs settle back into their habitual state of breathing, and then try the exercise again.

If this exercise is repeated three times in succession with quiet care, its effect will be very evident in the refreshment felt when a woman begins sewing again.

At the very most it can only take two minutes to go through the whole exercise and be ready to repeat it.

That will mean six minutes for the three successive times.

Six minutes can easily be made up by the renewed vigor that comes from the long breath and change of attitude. Stopping for the exercise three times a day will only take eighteen—or at the most twenty-minutes out of the day's work and it will put much more than that into the work in new power.

Third—We must remember that we need not sew in a badly cramped position. Of course the exercises will help us out of the habitually cramped attitude, but we cannot expect them to help us so much unless we make an effort while sewing to be as little cramped as possible.

The exercises give us a new standard of erectness, and that new standard will make us sensitive to the wrong attitude.

We will constantly notice when our chests get cramped and settled down on our stomachs and by expanding them and lifting them, even as we sew, the healthy attitude will get to be second nature.

Fourth—We must sew with our hands and our arms, not with our spines, the backs of our necks, or our legs. The unnecessary strain she puts into her sewing makes a woman more tired than anything else. To avoid this she must get sensitive to the strain, and every time she perceives it drop it; consciously, with a decided use of her will, until she has established the habit of working without strain. The gentle raising of the head to the erect position after the breathing exercise will let out a great deal of strain, and so make us more sensitive to its return when we begin to sew, and the more sensitive we get to it the sooner we can drop it.

I think I hear a woman say, "I have neither the time nor the strength to attend to all this." My answer is, such exercise will save time and strength in the end.

CHAPTER XXIII

Do not Hurry

HOW can any one do anything well while in a constant state of rush? How can any one see anything clearly while in a constant state of rush? How can any one expect to keep healthy and strong while in a constant state of rush?

But most of my readers may say, "I am not in a constant state of rush—I only hurry now and then when I need to hurry."

The answer to that is "Prove it, prove it." Study yourself a little, and see whether you find yourself chronically in a hurry or not.

If you will observe yourself carefully with a desire to find the hurry tendency, and to find it thoroughly, in order to eliminate it, you will be surprised to see how much of it there is in you.

The trouble is that all our standards are low, and to raise our standards we must drop that which interferes with the most wholesome way of living.

As we get rid of all the grosser forms of hurry we find in ourselves other hurry habits that are finer and more subtle, and gradually our standards of quiet, deliberate ways get higher; we become more sensitive to hurry, and a hurried way of doing things grows more and more disagreeable to us.

Watch the women coming out of a factory in the dinner hour or at six o'clock. They are almost tumbling over each other in their hurry to get away. They are putting on their jackets, pushing in their hatpins, and running along as if their dinner were running away from them.

Something akin to that same attitude of rush we can see in any large city when the clerks come out of the shops, for their luncheon hour, or when the work of the day is over.

If we were to calculate in round numbers the amount of time saved by this rush to get away from the shop, we should find three minutes, probably the maximum—and if we balance that against the loss to body and mind which is incurred, we should find the three minutes' gain quite overweighted by the loss of many hours, perhaps days, because of the illness which must be the result of such habitual contraction.

It is safe to predict when we see a woman rushing away from factory or shop that she is not going to "let up" on that rate of speed until she is back again at work. Indeed, having once started brain and body with such an exaggerated impetus, it is not possible to quiet down without a direct and decided use of the will, and how is that decided action to be taken if the brain is so befogged with the habit of hurry that it knows no better standard?

One of the girls from a large factory came rushing up to the kind, motherly head of the boarding house the other day saying:—

"It is abominable that I should be kept waiting so long for my dinner. I have had my first course and here I have been waiting twenty minutes for my dessert."

The woman addressed looked up quietly to the clock and saw that it was ten minutes past twelve.

"What time did you come in?" she said. "At twelve o'clock."

"And you have had your first course?"

"Yes."

"And waited twenty minutes for your dessert?"

"Yes!" (snappishly).

"How can that be when you came in at twelve o'clock, and it is now only ten minutes past?"

Of course there was nothing to say in answer, but whether the girl took it to heart and so raised her standard of quiet one little bit, I do not know.

One can deposit a fearful amount of strain in the brain with only a few moments' impatience.

I use the word "fearful" advisedly, for when the strain is once deposited it is not easily removed, especially when every day and every moment of every day is adding to the strain.

The strain of hurry makes contractions in brain and body with which it is impossible to work freely and easily or to accomplish as much as might be done without such contractions.

The strain of hurry befogs the brain so that it is impossible for it to expand to an unprejudiced point of view.

The strain of hurry so contracts the whole nervous and muscular systems that the body can take neither the nourishment of food nor of fresh air as it should.

There are many women who work for a living, and women who do not work for a living, who feel hurried from morning until they go to bed at night, and they must, perforce, hurry to sleep and hurry awake.

Often the day seems so full, and one is so pressed for time that it is impossible to get in all there is to do, and yet a little quiet thinking will show that the important things can be easily put into two thirds of the day, and the remaining third is free for rest, or play, or both.

Then again, there is real delight in quietly fitting one thing in after another when the day must be full, and the result at the end of the day is only healthy fatigue from which a good night's rest will refresh us entirely.

There is one thing that is very evident—a feeling of hurry retards our work, it does not hasten it, and the more quietly we can do what is before us, the more quickly and vigorously we do it.

The first necessity is to find ourselves out—to find out for a fact when we do hurry, and how we hurry, and how we have the sense of hurry with us all the time. Having willingly, and gladly, found ourselves out, the remedy is straight before us.

Nature is on the side of leisure and will come to our aid with higher standards of quiet, the possibilities of which are always in every one's brain, if we only look to find them.

To sit five minutes quietly taking long breaths to get a sense of leisure every day will be of very great help—and then when we find ourselves hurrying, let us stop and recall the best quiet we know—that need only take a few seconds, and the gain is sure to follow.

Festina lente (hasten slowly) should be in the back of our brains all day and every day.

> "'T is haste makes waste, the sage avers,
> And instances are far too plenty;
> Whene'er the hasty impulse stirs,
> Put on the brake, Festina Lente."

CHAPTER XXIV

The Care of an Invalid

TO take really good care of one who is ill requires not only knowledge but intelligent patience and immeasurable tact.

A little knowledge will go a great way, and we do not need to be trained nurses in order to help our friends to bear their illnesses patiently and quietly and to adjust things about them so that they are enabled to get well faster because of the care we give them.

Sometimes if we have only fifteen minutes in the morning and fifteen minutes at night to be with a sick friend, we can so arrange things for the day and for the night that we will have left behind us a directly curative influence because our invalid feels cared for in the best way, and has confidence enough to follow the suggestions we have given.

More depends upon the spirit with which we approach an invalid than anything else.

A trained nurse who has graduated at the head of her class and has executive ability, who knows exactly what to do and when to do it, may yet bring such a spirit of self-importance and bustle that everything she does for the invalid's ease, comfort, and recuperation is counteracted by the unrestful "professional" spirit with which the work is done.

On the other hand, a woman who has only a slight knowledge of nursing can bring so restful and unobtrusive an atmosphere with her that the invalid gains from her very presence.

Overwhelming kindness is not only tiresome and often annoying, but a serious drag on one who is ill.

People who are so busy doing kindnesses seldom consult the invalid's preferences at all. They are too full of their own selfish kindliness and self-importance.

I remember a woman who was suffering intensely from neuralgia in her face. A friend, proud of the idea of caring for her and giving up her own pleasure to stay in the darkened room and keep the sufferer's face bathed in hot water, made such a rustling back and forth with her skirts in getting the water that the strain of the constant noise and movement not only counteracted any relief that might have come from the heat, but it increased the pain and made the nervous condition of the patient much worse.

So it is with a hundred and one little "kindnesses" that people try to do for others when they are ill.

They talk to amuse them when the invalids would give all in their power to have a little quiet.

They sit like lumps and say nothing when a little light, easy chatting might divert the invalid's attention and so start up a gentle circulation which would tend directly toward health.

Or, they talk and are entertaining for a while in a very helpful way, but not knowing when to stop, finally make the patient so tired that they undo all the good of the first fifteen minutes.

They flood the room with light, "to make it look pleasant," when the invalid longs for the rest of a darkened room; or they draw the shades when the patient longs for the cheerfulness of sunlight.

They fuss and move about to do this or that and the other "kindness" when the sick person longs for absolute quiet.

They shower attentions when the first thing that is desired is to be let alone. One secret of the whole trouble in this oppressive care of the sick is that this sort of caretaker is interested more to please herself and feel the satisfaction of her own benefactions than she is to really please the friend for whom she is caring. Another trouble is common ignorance. Some women would gladly sacrifice anything to help a friend to get well; they would give their time and their strength gladly and count it as nothing, but they do not know how to care for the sick. Often such people are sadly discouraged because they see that they are only bringing discomfort where, with all their hearts, they desire to bring comfort. The first necessity in the right care for the sick is to be quiet and cheerful. The next is to aim, without disturbing the invalid, to get as true an idea as possible of the condition necessary to help the patient to get well. The third is to bring about those conditions with the least possible amount of friction.

Find out what the invalid likes and how she likes it by observation and not by questions.

Sometimes, of course, a question must be asked. If we receive a snappish answer, let us not resent it, but blame the illness and be grateful if, along with the snappishness, we find out what suits our patient best.

If we see her increasing her pain by contracting and giving all her attention to complaining, we cannot help her by telling her that that sort of thing is not going to make her well. But we can soothe her in a way that will enable her to see it for herself.

Often the right suggestion, no matter how good it is, will only annoy the patient and send her farther on in the wrong path; but if given in some gentle roundabout way, so that she feels that she has discovered for herself what you have been trying to tell her, it will work wonders toward her recovery.

If you want to care for the sick in a way that will truly help them toward recovery, you must observe and study,— study and observe, and never resent their irritability.

See that they have the right amount of air; that they have the right nourishment at the right intervals. Let them have things their own way, and done in their own way so far as is possible without interfering with what is necessary to their health.

Remember that there are times when it is better to risk deferring recovery a little rather than force upon an invalid what is not wanted, especially when it is evident that resistance will be harmful.

Quiet, cheerfulness, light, air, nourishment, orderly surroundings, and to be let judiciously alone; those are the conditions which the amateur nurse must further, according to her own judgment and, her knowledge of the friend she is nursing.

For this purpose she must, as I have said, study and observe, and observe and study.

I do not mean necessarily to do all this when she is "off duty," but to so concentrate when she is attending to the wants of her friend that every moment and every thought will be used to the best gain of the patient herself, and not toward our ideas of her best gain.

A little careful effort of this kind will open a new and interesting vista to the nurse as well as the patient.

CHAPTER XXV

The Habit of Illness

IT is surprising how many invalids there are who have got well and do not know it! When you feel ill and days drag on with one ill feeling following another, it is not a pleasant thing to be told that you are quite well. Who could be expected to believe it? I should like to know how many men and women there are who will read this article, who are well and do not know it; and how many of such men and women will take the hint I want to give them and turn honestly toward finding themselves out in a way that will enable them to discover and acknowledge the truth?

Nerves form habits. They actually form habits in themselves. If a woman has had an organic trouble which has caused certain forms of nervous discomfort, when the organic trouble is cured the nerves are apt to go on for a time with the same uncomfortable feelings because during the period of illness they had formed the habit of such discomfort. Then is the time when the will must be used to overcome such habits. The trouble is that when the doctor tells these victims of nervous habit that they are really well they will not believe him. "How can I be well," they say, "when I suffer just as I did while I was ill?" If then the doctor is fortunate enough to convince them of the fact that it is only the nervous habit formed from their illness which causes them to suffer, and that they can rouse their wills to overcome intelligently this habit, then they can be well in a few weeks when they might have been apparently ill for many months—or perhaps even years.

Nerves form the habit of being tired. A woman can get very much overfatigued at one time and have the impression of the fatigue so strongly on her nerves that the next time she is only a little tired she will believe she is very tired, and so her life will go until the habit of being tired has been formed in her nerves and she believes that she is tired all the time—whereas if the truth were known she might easily feel rested all the time.

It is often very difficult to overcome the habit which the nerves form as a result of an attack of nervous prostration. It is equally hard to convince any one getting out of such an illness that the habit of his nerves tries to make him believe he cannot do a little more every day—when he really can, and would be better for it. Many cases of nervous prostration which last for years might be cured in as many months if the truth about nerve habits were recognized and acted upon.

Nerves can form bad habits and they can form good habits, but of all the bad habits formed by nerves perhaps the very worst is the habit of being ill. These bad habits of illness engender an unwillingness to let go of them. They seem so real. "I do not want to suffer like this," I hear an invalid say; "if it were merely a habit don't you think I would throw it off in a minute?"

I knew a young physician who had made somewhat of a local reputation in the care of nerves, and a man living in a far-distant country, who had been for some time a chronic invalid, happened by accident to hear of him. My friend was surprised to receive a letter from this man, offering to pay him the full amount of all fees he would earn in one month and as much more as he might ask if he would spend that time in the house with him and attempt his cure.

Always interested in new phases of nerves, and having no serious case on hand himself at the time, he assented and went with great interest on this long journey to, as he hoped, cure one man. When he arrived he found his patient most charming. He listened attentively to the account of his years of illness, inquired of others in the house with him, and then went to bed and to sleep. In the morning he woke with a sense of unexplained depression. In searching about for the cause he went over his interviews of the day before and found a doubt in his mind which he would hardly acknowledge; but by the end of the next day he said to himself: "What a fool I was to come so far without a more complete knowledge of what I was coming to! This man has been well for years and does not know it. It is the old habit of his illness that is on him; the illness itself must have left him ten years ago."

The next day—the first thing after breakfast—he took a long walk in order to make up his mind what to do, and finally decided that he had engaged to stay one month and must keep to his promise. It would not do to tell the invalid the truth—the poor man would not believe it. He was self-willed and self-centered, and his pains and discomforts, which came simply from old habits of illness, were as real to him as if they had been genuine. Several physicians had emphasized his belief that he was ill. One doctor—so my friend was told—who saw clearly the truth of the case, ventured to hint at it and was at once discharged. My friend knew all these difficulties and, when he made up his mind that the only right thing for him to do was to stay, he found himself intensely interested in trying to approach his patient with so much delicacy that he could finally convince him of the truth; and I am happy to say that his efforts were to a great degree successful. The patient was awakened to the fact that, if he tried, he could be a well man. He never got so far as to see that he really was a well man who was allowing old habits to keep him ill; but he got enough of a new and healthy point of view to improve greatly and to feel a hearty sense of gratitude toward the man who had enlightened him. The long habit of illness had dulled his brain too much for him to appreciate the whole truth about himself.

The only way that such an invalid's brain can be enlightened is by going to work very gently and leading him to the light—never by combating. This young physician whom I mention was successful only through making friends with his patient and leading him gradually to appear to discover for himself the fact which all the time the physician was really telling him. The only way to help others is to help them to help themselves, and this is especially the truth with nerves.

If you, my friend, are so fortunate as to find out that your illness is more a habit of illness than illness itself, do not expect to break the habit at once. Go about it slowly and with common sense. A habit can be broken sooner than it can be formed, but even then it cannot be broken immediately. First recognize that your uncomfortable feelings whether of eyes, nose, stomach, back of neck, top of head, or whatever it may be, are mere habits, and then go about gradually but steadily ignoring them. When once you find that your own healthy self can assert itself and realize that you are stronger than your habits, these habits of illness will weaken and finally disappear altogether.

The moment an illness gets hold of one, the illness has the floor, so to speak, and the temptation is to consider it the master of the situation—and yielding to this temptation is the most effectual way of beginning to establish the habits which the illness has started, and makes it more difficult to know when one is well. On the other hand it is clearly possible to yield completely to an illness and let Nature take its course, and at the same time to take a mental attitude of wholesomeness toward it which will deprive the illness of much of its power. Nature always tends toward health; so we have the working of natural law entirely on our side. If the attitude of a man's mind is healthy, when he gets well he is well. He is not bothered long with the habits of his illness, for he has never allowed them to gain any hold upon him. He has neutralized the effect of the would be habits in the beginning so that they could not get a firm hold. We can counteract bad habits with good ones any time that we want to if we only go to work in the right way and are intelligently persistent.

It would be funny if it were not sad to hear a man say, "Well, you know I had such and such an illness years ago and I never really recovered from the effects of it," and to know at the same time that he had kept himself in the effects of it, or rather the habits of his nerves had kept him there, and he had been either ignorant or unwilling to use his will to throw off those habits and gain the habits of health which were ready and waiting.

People who cheerfully turn their hearts and minds toward health have so much, so very much, in their favor.

Of course, there are laws of health to be learned and carefully followed in the work of throwing off habits of illness. We must rest; take food that is nourishing, exercise, plenty of sleep and fresh air—yet always with the sense that the illness is only something to get rid of, and our own healthy attitude toward the illness is of the greatest importance.

Sometimes a man can go right ahead with his work, allow an illness to run its course, and get well without interrupting his work in the least, because of his strong aim toward health which keeps his illness subordinate. But this is not often the case. An illness, even though it be treated as subordinate, must be respected more or less according to its nature. But when that is done normally no bad habits will be left behind.

I know a young girl who was ill with strained nerves that showed themselves in weak eyes and a contracted stomach. She is well now—entirely well—but whenever she gets a little tired the old habits of eyes and stomach assert themselves, and she holds firmly on to them, whereas each time of getting overtired might be an opportunity to break up these evil habits by a right amount of rest and a healthy amount of ignoring.

This matter of habit is a very painful thing when it is supported by inherited tendencies. If a young person overdoes and gets pulled down with fatigue the fatigue expresses itself in the weakest part of his body. It may be in the stomach and consequently appear as indigestion; it may be in the head and so bring about severe headaches, and it may be in both stomach and head.

If it is known that such tendencies are inherited the first thought that almost inevitably comes to the mind is: "My father always had headaches and my grandfather, too. Of course, I must expect them now for the rest of my life." That thought interpreted rightly is: "My grandfather formed the headache habit, my father inherited the habit and clinched it—now, of course, I must expect to inherit it, and I will do my best to see if I cannot hold on to the habit as well as they did—even better, because I can add my own hold to that which I have inherited from both my ancestors."

Now, of course, a habit of illness, whether it be of the head, stomach, or of both, is much more difficult to discard when it is inherited than when it is first acquired in a personal illness of our own; but, because it is difficult, it is none the less possible to discard it, and when the work has been accomplished the strength gained from the steady, intelligent effort fully compensates for the difficulty of the task.

One must not get impatient with a bad habit in one's self; it has a certain power while it lasts, and can acquire a very strong hold. Little by little it must be dealt with—patiently and steadily. Sometimes it seems almost as if such habits had intelligence—for the more you ignore them the more rampant they become, and there is a Rubicon to cross, in the process of ignoring which, when once passed, makes the work of gaining freedom easier; for when the backbone of the habit is broken it weakens and seems to fade away of itself, and we awaken some fine morning and it has gone—really gone.

Many persons are in a prison of bad habits simply because they do not know how to get out—not because they do not want to get out. If we want to help a friend out of the habit of illness it is most important first to be sure that it is a habit, and then to remember that a suggestion is seldom responded to unless it is given with generous sympathy and love. Indeed, when a suggestion is given with lack of sympathy or with contempt the tendency is to make the invalid turn painfully away from the speaker and hug her bad habits more closely to herself. What we can do, however, is to throw out a suggestion here and there which may lead such a one to discover the truth for herself; then, if she comes to you with sincere interest in her discovery, don't say: "Yes, I have thought so for some time." Keep yourself out of it, except in so far as you can give aid which is really wanted, and accepted and used.

Beware of saying or doing anything to or for any one which will only rouse resentment and serve to push deeper into the brain an impression already made by a mistaken conviction. More than half of the functional and nervous illnesses in the world are caused by bad habit, either formed or inherited.

Happy are those who discover the fact for themselves and, with the intelligence born from such discovery, work with patient insight until they have freed themselves from bondage. Happy are those who feel willing to change any mistaken conviction or prejudice and to recognize it as a sin against the truth.

CHAPTER XXVI

What is It that Makes Me so Nervous?

THE two main reasons why women are nervous are, first, that they do not take intelligent care of their bodies, and secondly, that they do not govern their emotions.

I know a woman who prefers to make herself genuinely miserable rather than take food normally, to eat it normally, and to exercise in the fresh air.

"Everybody is against me," she says; and if you answer her, "My dear, you are acting against yourself by keeping your stomach on a steady strain with too much unmasticated, unhealthy, undigested food," she turns a woebegone face on you and asks how you can be "so material."

"Nobody loves me; nobody is kind to me. Everybody neglects me," she says.

And when you answer, "How can any one love you when you are always whining and complaining? How can any one be kind to you when you resent and resist every friendly attention because it does not suit your especial taste? Indeed, how can you expect anything from any one when you are giving nothing yourself?" She replies,

"But I am so nervous. I suffer. Why don't they sympathize?"

"My dear child, would you sympathize with a woman who went down into the cellar and cried because she was so cold, when fresh air and warm sunshine were waiting for her outside?"

This very woman herself is cold all the time. She piles covers over herself at night so that the weight alone would be enough to make her ill. She sleeps with the heat turned on in her room. She complains all day of cold when not complaining of other things. She puts such a strain on her stomach that it takes all of her vitality to look after her food; therefore she has no vitality left with which to resist the cold. Of course she resists the idea of a good brisk walk in the fresh air, and yet, if she took the walk and enjoyed it, it would start up her circulation, give her blood more oxygen, and help her stomach to go through all its useless labor better.

When a woman disobeys all the laws of nervous health how can she expect not to have her nerves rebel? Nerves in themselves are exquisitely sensitive—with a direct tendency toward health.

"Don't give me such unnecessary work," the stomach cries. "Don't stuff me full of the wrong things. Don't put a bulk of food into me, but chew your food, so that I shall not have to do my own work and yours, too, when the food gets down here."

And there is the poor stomach, a big nervous centre in close communication with the brain, protesting and protesting, and its owner interprets all these protestations into: "I am so unhappy. I have to work so much harder than I ought. Nobody loves me. Oh, why am I so nervous?"

The blood also cries out: "Give me more oxygen. I cannot help the lungs or the stomach or the brain to do their work properly unless you take exercise in the fresh air that will feed me truly and send me over the body with good, wholesome vigor."

Now there is another thing that is sadly evident about the young woman who will not take fresh air, nor eat the right food, nor masticate properly the food that she does eat. When she goes out for a walk she seems to fight the fresh air; she walks along full of resistance and contraction, and tightens all her muscles so that she moves as if she were tied together with ropes. The expression of her face is one of miserable strain and endurance; the tone of her voice is full of complaint. In eating either she takes her food with the appearance of hungry grabbing, or she refuses it with a fastidious scorn. Any nervous woman who really wants to find herself out, in order to get well and strong, and contented and happy, will see in this description a reflection of herself, even though it may be an exaggerated reflection.

Did you ever see a tired, hungry baby fight his food? His mother tries to put the bottle to his mouth, and the baby cries and cries, and turns his head away, and brandishes his little arms about, as if his mother were offering him something bitter. Then, finally, when his mother succeeds in getting him to open his mouth and take the food it makes you smile all over to see the contrast: he looks so quiet and contented, and you can see his whole little body expand with satisfaction.

It is just the same inherited tendency in a nervous woman that makes her either consciously or unconsciously fight exercise and fresh air, fight good food and eating it rightly, fight everything that is wholesome and strengthening and quieting to her nerves, and cling with painful tenacity to everything that is contracting and weakening, and productive of chronic strain.

There is another thing that a woman fights: she fights rest. Who has not seen a tired woman work harder and harder, when she was tired, until she has worn herself to a state of nervous irritability and finally has to succumb for want of strength? Who has not seen this same tired woman, the moment she gets back a little grain of strength, use it up again at once instead of waiting until she had paid back her principal and could use only the interest of her strength while keeping a good balance in reserve?

"I wish my mother would not do so many unnecessary things," said an anxious daughter.

A few days after this the mother came in tired, and, with a fagged look on her face and a fagged tone in her voice, said: "Before I sit down I must go and see poor Mrs. Robinson. I have just heard that she has been taken ill with nervous prostration. Poor thing! Why couldn't she have taken care of herself?"

"But, mother," her daughter answered, "I have been to see Mrs. Robinson, and taken her some flowers, and told her how sorry you would be to hear that she was ill."

"My dear," said the fagged mother with a slight tone of irritation in her voice, "that was very good of you, but of course that was not my going, and if I should let to-day pass without going to see her, when I have just heard of her illness, it would be unfriendly and unneighborly and I should not forgive myself."

"But, mother, you are tired; you do need to rest so much."

"My dear," said the mother with an air of conscious virtue, "I am never too tired to do a neighborly kindness."

When she left the house her daughter burst into tears and let out the strain which had been accumulating for weeks.

Finally, when she had let down enough to feel a relief, a funny little smile came through the tears.

"There is one nervously worn-out woman gone to comfort and lift up another nervously worn-out woman—if that is not the blind leading the blind then I don't know. I wonder how long it will be before mamma, too, is in the ditch?"

This same story could be reversed with the mother in the daughter's place, and the daughter in the mother's. And, indeed, we see slight illustrations of it, in one way or the other, in many families and among many friends.

This, then, is the first answer to any woman's question, "Why am I so nervous?" Because you do not use common sense in taking exercise, fresh air, nourishment, and rest.

Nature tends toward health. Your whole physical organism tends toward health. If you once find yourself out and begin to be sensible you will find a great, vigorous power carrying you along, and you will be surprised to see how fast you gain. It may be some time before Nature gets her own way with you entirely, because when one has been off the track for long it must take time to readjust; but when we begin to go with the laws of health, instead of against them, we get into a healthy current and gain faster than would have seemed possible when we were outside of it, habitually trying to oppose the stream.

The second reason why women are nervous is that they do not govern their emotions. Very often it is the strain of unpleasant emotions that keeps women nervous, and when we come really to understand we find that the strain is there because the woman does not get her own way. She has not money enough.

She has to live with some one she dislikes. She feels that people do not like her and are neglectful of her. She believes that she has too much work to do. She wishes that she had more beauty in her life.

Sometimes a woman is entirely conscious of when or why she fails to get her own way; then she knows what she is fretting about, and she may even know that the fretting is a strain that keeps her tired and nervously irritated. Sometimes a woman is entirely unconscious of what it is that is keeping her in a chronic state of nervous irritability. I have seen a woman express herself as entirely resigned to the very circumstance or person that she was unconsciously resisting so fiercely that her resistance kept her ill half of the time. In such cases the strain is double. First, there is the strain of the person or circumstance chronically resisted and secondly, there is the strain of the pose of saintly resignation. It is bad enough to pose to other people, but when we pose to other people and to ourselves too the strain is twice as bad.

Imagine a nerve specialist saying to his patient, "My dear madam, you really must stop being a hypocrite. You have not the nervous strength to spare for it." In most cases, I fear, the woman would turn on him indignantly and go home to be more of a hypocrite than ever, and so more nervously ill.

I have seen a woman cry and make no end of trouble because she had to have a certain relative live in the house with her, simply because her relative "got on her nerves." Then, after the relative had left the house, this same woman cried and still kept on making no end of trouble because she thought she had done wrong in sending "Cousin Sophia" away; and the poor, innocent, uncomplaining victim was brought back again. Yet it never seemed to occur to the nervous woman that "Cousin Sophia" was harmless, and that her trouble came entirely from the way in which she constantly resented and resisted little unpolished ways.

I do not know how many times "Cousin Sophia" may be sent off and brought back again; nor how many times other things in my nervous friend's life may have to be pulled to pieces and then put together again, for she has not yet discovered that the cause of the nervous trouble is entirely in herself, and that if she would stop resisting "Cousin Sophia's" innocent peculiarities, stop resisting other various phases of her life that do not suit her, and begin to use her will to yield where she has always resisted, her load would be steadily and happily lifted.

The nervous strain of doing right is very painful; especially so because most women who are under this strain do not really care about doing right at all. I have seen a woman quibble and talk and worry about what she believed to be a matter of right and wrong in a few cents, and then neglect for months to pay a poor man a certain large amount of money which he had honestly earned, and which she knew he needed.

The nervous conscience is really no conscience at all. I have seen a woman worry over what she owed to a certain other woman in the way of kindness, and go to a great deal of trouble to make her kindness complete; and then, on the same day, show such hard, unfeeling cruelty toward another friend that she wounded her deeply, and that without a regret.

A nervous woman's emotions are constantly side-tracking her away from the main cause of her difficulty, and so keeping her nervous. A nervous woman's desire to get her own way—and strained rebellion at not getting her own way—bedazzles or befogs her brain so that her nerves twist off into all sorts of emotions which have nothing whatever to do with the main cause. The woman with the troublesome relative wants to be considered good and kind and generous. The woman with the nervous money conscience wants to be considered upright and just in her dealings with others. All women with various expressions of nervous conscience want to ease their consciences for the sake of their own comfort—not in the least for the sake of doing right.

I write first of the nervous hypocrite because in her case the nervous strain is deeper in and more difficult to find. To watch such a woman is like seeing her in a terrible nightmare, which she steadily "sugar-coats" by her complacent belief in her own goodness. If, among a thousand nervous "saints" who may read these words, one is thereby enabled to find herself out, they are worth the pains of writing many times over. The nervous hypocrites who do not find themselves out get sicker and sicker, until finally they seem to be of no use except to discipline those who have the care of them.

The greatest trouble comes through the befogging emotions. A woman begins to feel a nervous strain, and that strain results in exciting emotions; these emotions again breed more emotions until she becomes a simmering mass of exciting and painful emotions which can be aroused to a boiling point at any moment by anything or any one who may touch a sensitive point. When a woman's emotions are aroused, and she is allowing herself to be governed by them, reason is out of the question, and any one who imagines that a woman can be made to understand common sense in a state like that will find himself entirely mistaken.

The only cure is for the woman herself to learn first how entirely impervious to common sense she is when she is in the midst of an emotional nerve storm, so that she will say, "Don't try to talk to me now; I am not reasonable, wait until I get quiet." Then, if she will go off by herself and drop her emotions, and also the strain behind her emotions, she will often come to a good, clear judgment without outside help; or, if not, she will come to the point where she will be ready and grateful to receive help from a clearer mind than her own.

"For goodness' sake, don't tell that to Alice," a young fellow said of his sister. "She will have fits first, and then indigestion and insomnia for six weeks." The lad was not a nerve specialist; neither was he interested in nerves—except to get away from them; but he spoke truly from common sense and his own experience with his sister.

The point is, to drop the emotions and face the facts. If nervous women would see the necessity for that, and would practice it, it would be surprising to see how their nerves would improve.

I once knew a woman who discovered that her emotions were running away with her and making her nervously ill. She at once went to work with a will, and every time something happened to rouse this great emotional wave she would deliberately force herself to relax and relax until the wave had passed over her and she could see things in a sensible light. When she was unable to go off by herself and lie down to relax, she would walk with her mind bent on making her feet feel heavy. When you drop the tension of the emotion, the emotion has nothing to hold on to and it must go.

I knew another woman who did not know how to relax; so, to get free from this emotional excitement, she would turn her attention at once to figures, to her personal accounts or even to saying the multiplication table. The steady concentration of her mind on dry figures and on "getting her sums right" left the rest of her brain free to drop its excitement and get into a normal state again.

Again it is sometimes owing to the pleasant emotions which some women indulge in to such an extreme that they are made ill. How many times have we heard of women who were "worn to a shred" by the delight of an opera, or a concert, or an exciting play? If these women only knew it, their pleasure would be far keener if they would let the enjoyment pass through them, instead of tightening up in their nerves and trying to hold on to it.

Nature in us always tends toward health, and toward pleasant sensations. If we relax out of painful emotions we find good judgment and happy instincts behind them. If we relax so that pleasant emotions can pass over our nerves they leave a deposit of happy sensation behind, which only adds to the store that Nature has provided for us.

To sum up: The two main reasons why women are nervous are that they do not take intelligent care of their bodies, and that they do not govern their emotions; but back of these reasons is the fact that they want their own way altogether too much. Even if a woman's own way is right, she has no business to push for it selfishly. If any woman thinks, "I could take intelligent care of my own body if I did not have to work so hard, or have this or that interference," let her go to work with her mind well armed to do what she can, and she will soon find that there are many ways in which she can improve in the normal care of her body, in spite of all the work and all the interferences.

To adapt an old saying, the women who are overworked and clogged with real interferences should aim to be healthy; and, if they cannot be healthy, then they should be as healthy as they can.

CHAPTER XXVII

Positive and Negative Effort

DID you ever have the grip? If you ever have you may know how truly it is named and how it does actually grip you so that it seems as if there were nothing else in the world at the time—it appears to entirely possess you. As the Irishman says, the grip is "the disease that lasts fur a week and it takes yer six weeks ter get over it." That is because it has possessed you so thoroughly that it must be routed out of every little fiber in your body before you are yourself again, and there are hidden corners where it lurks and hides, and it often has to be actually pulled out of them. Now it has been already recognized that if we relax and do not resist a severe cold it leaves us open so that our natural circulation carries away the cold much more quickly than if we allowed ourselves to be full of resistance to the discomfort and the consequent physical contraction that impeded the circulation and holds the cold in our system.

My point is this—that it is comparatively easy to relax out of a cold. We can do it with only a negative effort, but to relax so that nature in her steady and unswerving tendency toward health can lift us out of the grip is quite another matter. When we feel ourselves entirely in the power of such a monster as that is at its worst, it is only by a very strong and positive effort of the will that we can yield so that nature can guide us into health, and we do not need the six weeks of getting well.

In order to gain this positive sense of yielding away from the disease rather than of letting it hold us, we must do what seems at the time the impossible—we must refuse to give our attention to the pain or discomfort and insist upon giving our attention entirely to yielding out of the contractions which the painful discomforts cause. In other words, we must give up resisting the grip. It is the same with any other disease or any pain. If we have the toothache and give all our attention to the toothache, it inevitably makes it worse; but if we give our attention to yielding out of the toothache contractions, it eases the pain even though it may be that only the dentist can stop it. Once I had an ulcerated tooth which lasted for a week. I had to yield so steadily to do my work during the day and to be able to sleep at all at night that it not only made the pain bearable, but when the tooth got well I was surprised to find how many habitual contractions I had dropped and how much more freedom of action I had before my tooth began to ulcerate. I should not wish to have another ulcerated tooth in order that I might gain more freedom, but I should wish to take every pain of body and mind so truly that when the pain was over I should have gained greater freedom than I had before it began.

You see it is the same with every pain and with every disease. Nature tends toward health and if we make the disease simply a reminder to yield—and to yield more deeply—and to put our positive effort there, we are opening the way for nature to do her best work. If our entire attention is given to yielding and we give no attention whatever to the pain, except as a reminder to yield, the result seems wonderful. It seems wonderful because so few of us have the habit of giving our entire attention to gaining our real freedom.

With most of us, the disease or discomfort is positive, and our effort against it is negative or no effort at all. A negative effort probably protects us from worse evil, but that is all; it does not seem to me that it can ever take us ahead, whereas a positive effort, while sometimes we seem to move upward in very slow stages, often takes us in great strides out of the enemy's country.

If we have the measles, the whooping cough, scarlet fever—even more serious diseases—and make the disease negative and our effort to free ourselves from it positive, the result is one thousand times worth while. And where the children have the measles and the whooping cough, and do not know how to help nature, the mothers can be positive for the children and make their measles and whooping cough negative. The positive attitude of a mother toward her sick child puts impatience or despair out of the question.

Do not think that I believe one can be positive all at once. We must work hard and insist over and over again before we can attain the positive attitude and having attained it, we have to lose it and gain it again, lose it and gain it again, many times before we get the habit of making all difficulties of mind and body negative, and our healthy attitude toward conquering them positive.

I said "difficulties of mind and body." I might better have said "difficulties of body, mind and character," or even character alone, for, after all, when you come to sift things down, it is the character that is at the root of all human life.

I know a woman who is constantly complaining. Every morning she has a series of pains to tell of, and her complaints spout out of her in a half-irritated, whining tone as naturally as she breathes. Over and over you think when you listen to her how useful all those pains of hers would be if she took them as a reminder to yield and in yielding to do her work better. But if one should venture to suggest such a possibility, it would only increase the complaints by one more—that of having unsympathetic friends and being misunderstood. "Nobody understands me—nobody understands me." How often we hear that complaint. How often in hearing it we make the mental question, "Do you understand yourself?"

You see the greatest impediment to our understanding ourselves is our unwillingness to see what is not good in ourselves. It is easy enough in a self-righteous attitude of what we believe to be humility to find fault with ourselves, but quite another thing when others find fault with us. When we are giving our attention to discomforts and pains in a way to give them positive power, and some one suggests that we might change our aim, then the resistance and resentment that are roused in us are very indicative of just where we are in our character.

Another strong indication of allowing our weaknesses and faults to be positive and our effort against them negative is the destructive habit of giving excuses. If fault is found with us and there is justice in it, it does not make the slightest difference how many things we have done that are good, or how much better we do than some one else does—the positive way is to say "thank you" in spirit and in words, and to aim directly toward freeing ourselves from the fault. How ridiculous it would seem if when we were told that we had a smooch on our left cheek, we were to insist vehemently upon the cleanliness of our right cheek, or our forehead, or our hands, instead of being grateful that our attention should be called to the smooch and taking soap and water and at once washing it off. Or how equally absurd it would be if we went into long explanations as to how the smooch would not have been there if it had not been for so and so, and so and so, or so and so,—and then with all our excuses and explanations and protestations, we let the smooch stay—and never really wash it off.

And yet this is not an exaggeration of what most of us do when our attention is called to defects of character. When we excuse and explain and tell how clean the other side of our face is, we are putting ourselves positively on the side of the smooch. So we are putting ourselves entirely on the side of the illness or the pain or the oppression of difficult circumstances when we give excuses or resist or pretend not to see fault in ourselves, or when we confess faults and are contented about them, or when we give all our attention to what is disagreeable and no attention to the normal way of gaining our health or our freedom.

Then all these expressions of self or of illness are to us positive, and our efforts against them only negative. In such cases, of course, the self possesses us as surely as the grip possesses us when we succumb entirely to all its horrors and make no positive effort to yield out of it. And the possession of the self is much worse, much deeper, much more subtle. When possessed with selfishness, we are laying up in our subconsciousness any number of self-seeking motives which come to the surface disguised and compel us to make impulsive and often foolish efforts to gain our own ends. The self is every day proving to be the enemy of the man or woman whom it possesses.

God leaves us free to obey Him or to choose our own selfish way, and in His infinite Providence He is constantly showing us that our own selfish way leads to death and obedience to Him leads to life. That is, that only in obedience to Him do we find our real freedom. He is constantly showering us with a tender generosity and kindness that seems inconceivable, and sometimes it seems as if more often than not we were refusing to see. Indeed we blind ourselves by making all pains of body and faults of soul positive and our efforts against them negative.

If we had a disagreeable habit which we wanted to conquer and asked a friend to remind us with a pinch every time he saw the habit, wouldn't it seem very strange if when he pinched us, according to agreement, we jumped and turned on him, rubbing our arm with indignation that he should have pinched? Or would it not be even funnier if we made the pinch merely a reminder to go on with the habit?

The Lord is pinching us in that way all the time, and we respond by being indignant at or complaining at our fate, or reply by going more deeply into our weaknesses of character by allowing them to be positive and the pinches only to emphasize them to us.

One trouble is that we do not recognize that there is an agreement between us and the Lord, or that we recognize and then forget it; and yet there should be—there is—more than an agreement, there is a covenant. And the Lord is steadily, unswervingly doing His part, and we are constantly failing in ours. The Lord in His loving kindness pinches—that is, reminds us—and we in our stupid selfishness do not use His reminders.

As an example of making our faults positive and our effort to conquer them negative, one very common form is found in a woman I know, who has times of informing her friends quite seriously and with apparent regret of her very wrong attitudes of mind. She tells how selfish she is and she gives examples of the absolute selfishness of her thoughts when she is appearing to do unselfish things. She tells of her efforts to do better and confesses what she believes to be the absolute futility of her effort. At first I was quite taken in by these confessions, and attracted by what seemed to be a clear understanding of herself and her own motives, but after a little longer acquaintance with her, made the discovery, which was at first surprising to me, that her confessions of evil came just as much from conceit as if she had been standing at the mirror admiring her own beauty. Selfish satisfaction is often found quite as much in mental attitudes of grief as in sensations of joy. Finally this woman has recognized for herself the conceit in her contemplation of her faults, and that she has not only allowed them to be positive while her attitude against them is negative; she has actually nursed them and been positive herself with their positiveness. Her attitude against them was therefore more than ordinarily negative.

The more common way of being negative while we allow our various forms of selfishness to positively govern us is, first in bewailing a weakness seriously, but constantly looking at it and weeping over it, and in that way suggesting it over and over to our brains so that we are really hypnotizing ourselves with the fault and enforcing its expression when we think we are in the effort to conquer it. Such is our negative attitude.

Now if we are convinced that evil in ourselves has no power unless we give it power, that is the first step toward making our efforts positive and so negativing the evil. If we are convinced that evil in ourselves has not only no power but no importance unless we give it power, that is a step still farther in advance. The next step is to refuse to submit to it and refuse to resist it. That means a positive yielding away from it and a positive attention to doing our work as well as we can do it, whatever that work may be.

There is one way in which people suffer intensely through being negative and allowing their temptations to be positive, and that is in the question of inherited evil. "How can I ever amount to anything with such inheritances? If you could see my father and what he is, and know that I am his daughter, you would easily appreciate why I have no hope for myself," said a young woman, and she was perfectly sincere in believing that because of her inherited temptations her life must be worthless. It took time and gentle, intelligent reasoning to convince her that not only are no inherited forms of selfishness ours unless by indulging we make them ours, but that, through knowing our inheritances, we are forewarned and forearmed, and the strength we gain from positive effort to free ourselves fully compensates us for what we have suffered in oppression from them. Such is the loving kindness of our Creator.

This woman of whom I am writing awoke to the true meaning of the story of the man who asked, before he went with the Lord Jesus Christ, first to go back and bury his father. The Lord answered, "Let the dead bury their dead, and come thou and follow me." When we feel that we must be bound down by our inheritances, we are surely not letting the dead bury their dead.

And so let us study the whole question more carefully and learn the necessity of letting all that is sickness and all that is evil be negative to us and our efforts to conquer it be positive; in that way the illness and the evil become less than negative,—they gradually are removed and disappear.

Why, in the mere matter of being tired, if we refuse to let the impression of the fatigue be positive to us, and insist upon being positive ourselves in giving attention to the fact that now we are going to rest, we get rested in half the time,—in much less than half the time. Some people carry chronic fatigue with them because of their steady attention to fatigue.

"I am tired, yes, but *I am going to get rested!"* That is the sensible attitude of mind.

Nature tends toward health. As we realize that and give our attention to it positively, we come to admire and love the healthy working of the laws of nature, and to feel the vigor of interest in trying to obey them intelligently. Nature's laws are God's laws, and God's laws tend toward the health of the spirit in all matters of the spirit as surely as they tend toward health of body in all natural things. That is a truth that as we work to obey we grow to see and to love with deepening reverence, and then indeed we find that God's laws are all positive, and that the workings of self are only negative.

CHAPTER XXVIII

Human Dust

WHEN we face the matter squarely and give it careful thought, it seems to appear very plainly that the one thing most flagrantly in the way of the people of to-day living according to plain common sense—spiritual common sense as well as material—is the fact that we are all living in a chronic state of excitement. It is easy to prove this fact by seeing how soon most of us suffer from ennui when "there is not anything going on." It seems now as if the average man or woman whom we see would find it quite impossible to stop and do nothing—for an hour or more. "But," some one will say, "why should I stop and do nothing when I am as busy as I can be all day long, and have my time very happily full?" Or some one else may say, "How can I stop and do nothing when I am nearly crazy with work and must feel that it is being accomplished?"

Now the answer to that is, "Certainly you should not stop and do nothing when you are busy and happily busy;" or, "Although your work will go better if you do not get 'crazy' about it, there is no need of interrupting it or delaying it by stopping to do nothing—but *you should be able to stop and do nothing,* and to do it quietly and contentedly at any time when it might be required of you."

No man, woman, or child knows the power, the very great power, for work and play—there is with one who has in the background always the ability to stop and do nothing.

If we observe enough, carefully enough, and quietly enough, to get sensitive to it, we can see how every one about us is living in excitement. I have seen women with nothing important to do come down to breakfast in excitement, give their orders for the day as if they were about running for a fire; and the standard of all those about them is so low that no one notices what a human dust is stirred up by all this flutter over nothing.

A man told me not long ago that he got tired out for the day in walking to his office with a friend, because they both talked so intensely. And that is not an unusual experience. This chronic state of strain and excitement in everyday matters makes a mental atmosphere which is akin to what the material atmosphere would be if we were persistently kicking up a dust in the road every step we took. Every one seems to be stirring up his own especial and peculiar dust and adding it to every one else's especial and peculiar dust.

We are all mentally, morally and spiritually sneezing or choking with our own dust and the dust of other people. How is it possible for us to get any clear, all-round view of life so long as the dust stirring habit is on us? So far from being able to enlarge our horizon, we can get no horizon at all, and so no perspective until this human dust is laid. And there is just this one thing about it, that is a delight to think of: When we know how to live so that our own dust is laid, that very habit of life keeps us clear from the dust of other people. Not only that, but when we are free from dust ourselves, the dust that the other men are stirring up about us does not interfere with our view of them. We see the men through their dust and we see how the dust with which they are surrounding themselves befogs them and impedes their progress. From the place of no dust you can distinguish dust and see through it. From the place of dust you cannot distinguish anything clearly. Therefore, if one wishes to learn the standards of living according to plain common sense, for body, mind, and spirit, and to apply the principles of such standards practically to their every-day life, the first absolute necessity is to get quiet and to stay quiet long enough to lay the dust.

You may know the laws of right eating, of right breathing, of exercise, and rest—but in this dust of excitement in daily life such knowledge helps one very little. You constantly forget, and forget, and forget. Or, if in a moment of forced acknowledgment to the need of better living, you make up your mind that you will live according to sensible laws of hygiene, you go along pretty well for a few weeks, perhaps even months, and then as you feel better physically, you get whirled off into the excitement again, and before you know it you are in the dust with the rest of the world, and all because you had no background for your good resolutions. You never had found and you did not understand quiet.

Did you ever see a wise mother come into a noisy nursery where perhaps her own children were playing excitedly with several little companions, who had been invited in to spend a rainy afternoon? The mother sees all the children in a great state of excitement over their play, and two or three of them disagreeing over some foolish little matter, with their brains in such a state that the nursery is thick with infantile human dust. What does the wise mother do? Add dust of her own by scolding and fretting and fuming over the noise that the children are making? No—no indeed. She first gets all the children's attention in any happy way she can, one or two at a time, and then when she has their individual attention to a small degree, she gets their united attention by inviting their interest in being so quiet that they "can hear a pin drop." The children get keenly interested in listening. The first time they do not hear the pin drop because Johnnie or Mollie moved a little. Mother talks with interest of what a very delightful thing it is to be for a little while so quiet that we can hear a pin drop. The second time something interferes, and the third time the children have become so well focused on listening that the little delicate sound is heard distinctly, and they beg mother to try and see if they cannot hear it again. By this time the dust is laid in the nursery, and by changing the games a little, or telling them a story first, the mother is able to leave a nursery full of quiet, happy children.

Now if we, who would like to live happily and keep well, according to plain common sense, can put ourselves with intelligent humility in the place of these little children and study to be quiet, we will be working for that background which is never failing in its possibilities of increasing light and warmth and the expanse of outlook.

First with regard to a quiet body. Indigestion makes us unquiet, therefore we must eat only wholesome food, and not too much of it, and we must eat it quietly. Poor breathing and poor blood makes us unquiet, therefore we should learn to expand our lungs to their full extent in the fresh air and give the blood plenty of oxygen. Breathing also has a direct effect on the circulation and the brain, and when we breathe quietly and rhythmically, we are quieting the movement of our blood as well as opening the channels so that it can flow without interruption. We are also quieting our brain and so our whole nervous system.

Lack of exercise makes us unquiet, because exercise supplies the blood more fully with oxygen and prevents it from flowing sluggishly, a sluggish circulation straining the nervous system. It is therefore important to take regular exercise.

Want of rest especially makes us unquiet; therefore we should attend to it that we get—as far as possible—what rest we need, and take all the rest we get in the best way. We cannot expect to fulfill these conditions all at once, but we can aim steadily to do so, and by getting every day a stronger focus and a steadier aim we can gain so greatly in fulfilling the standards of a healthy mind in a healthy body, and so much of our individual dust will be laid, that I may fairly promise a happy astonishment at the view of life which will open before us, and the power for use and enjoyment that will come.

Let us see now how we would begin practically, having made up our minds to do all in our power to lay the dust and get a quiet background. We must begin in what may seem a very small way. It seems to be always the small beginnings that lead to large and solidly lasting results. Not only that, but when we begin in the small way and the right way to reach any goal, we can find no short cuts and no seven-league boots.

We must take every step and take it decidedly in order to really get there. We must place one brick and then another, exactly, and place every brick—to make a house that will stand.

But now for our first step toward laying the dust. Let us take half an hour every day and do nothing in it. For the first ten minutes we will probably be wretched, for the next ten minutes we may be more wretched, but for the last five minutes we will get a sense of quiet and at first the dust, although not laid, will cease to whirl. And then—an interesting fact—what seems to us quiet in the beginning of our attempt, will seem like noise and whirlwinds, after we have gone further along. Some one may easily say that it is absurd to take half an hour a day to do nothing in. Or that "Nature abhors a vacuum, and how is it possible to do nothing? Our minds will be thinking of or working on something."

In answer to this, I might say with the Irishman, "Be aisy, but if you can't be aisy, be as aisy as you can!" Do nothing as well as you can. When you begin thinking of anything, drop it. When you feel restless and as if you could not keep still another minute, relax and make yourself keep still. I should take many days of this insistence upon doing nothing and dropping everything from my mind before taking the next step. For to drop everything from one's mind, for half an hour is not by any means an easy matter. Our minds are full of interests, full of resistances. With some of us, our minds are full of resentment. And what we have to promise ourselves to do is for that one-half hour a day to take nothing into consideration. If something comes up that we are worrying about, refuse to consider it. If some resentment to a person or a circumstance comes to mind, refuse to consider it.

I know all this is easier to say than to do, but remember, please, that it is only for half an hour every day-only half an hour. Refuse to consider anything for half an hour. Having learned to sit still, or lie still, and think of nothing with a moderate degree of success, and with most people the success can only be moderate at best, the next step is to think quietly of taking long, gentle, easy breaths for half an hour. A long breath and then a rest, two long breaths and then a rest. One can quiet and soothe oneself inside quite wonderfully with the study of long gentle breaths. But it must be a study. We must study to begin inhaling gently, to change to the exhalation with equal delicacy, and to keep the same gentle, delicate pressure throughout, each time trying to make the breath a little longer.

After we have had many days of the gentle, long breaths at intervals for half an hour, then we can breathe rhythmically (inhale counting five or ten, exhale counting five or ten), steadily for half an hour, trying all the time to have the breath more quiet, gentle and steady, drawing it in and letting it out with always decreasing effort. It is wonderful when we discover how little effort we really need to take a full and vigorous breath. This half hour's breathing exercise every day will help us to the habit of breathing rhythmically all the time, and a steady rhythmic breath is a great physical help toward a quiet mind.

We can mingle with the deep breathing simple exercises of lifting each arm slowly and heavily from the shoulder, and then letting it drop a dead weight, and pausing while we feel conscious of our arms resting without tension in the lap or on the couch.

But all this has been with relation to the body, and it is the mental and moral dust of which I am writing. The physical work for quiet is only helpful as it makes the body a better instrument for the mind and for the will. A quiet body is of no use if it contains an unquiet mind which is going to pull it out of shape or start it up in agitation at the least provocation. In such a case, the quiet body in its passive state is only a more responsive instrument to the mind that wants to raise a dust. One—and the most helpful way of quieting the mind—is through a steady effort at concentration. One can concentrate; on doing nothing—that is, on sitting quietly in a chair or lying quietly on the bed or the floor. Be quiet, keep quiet, be quiet, keep quiet. That is the form of concentration, that is the way of learning to do nothing to advantage. Then we concentrate on the quiet breathing, to have it gentle, steady, and without strain. In the beginning we must take care to concentrate without strain, and without emotion, use our minds quietly, as one might watch a bird who was very near, to see what it will do next, and with care not to frighten it away.

These are the great secrets of true strengthening concentration. The first is dropping everything that interferes. The second is working to concentrate easily without emotion. They are really one and the same. If we work to drop everything that interferes, we are so constantly relaxing in order to concentrate that the very process drops strain bit by bit, little by little.

An unquiet mind, however, full of worries, anxieties, resistances, resentments, and full of all varieties of agitation, going over and over things to try to work out problems that are not in human hands, or complaining and fretting and puzzling because help seems to be out of human power, such a mind which is befogged and begrimed by the agitation of its own dust is not a cause in itself—it is an effect. The cause is the reaching and grasping, the unreasonable insistence on its own way of kicking, dust-raising self-will at the back of the mind.

A quiet will, a will that can remain quiet through all emergencies, is not a self-will. It is the self that raises the dust—the self that wants, and strains to get its own way, and turns and twists and writhes if it does not get its own way.

God's will is quiet. We see it in the growth of the trees and the flowers. We see it in the movement of the planets of the Universe. We see God's mind in the wonderful laws of natural science. Most of all we see and feel, when we get quiet ourselves, God's love in every thing and every one.

If we want the dust laid, we must work to get our bodies quiet. We must drop all that interferes with quiet in our minds, and we must give up wanting our own way. We must believe that God's way is immeasurably beyond us and that if we work quietly to obey Him, He will reveal to us His way in so far as we need to know it, and will prepare us for and guide us to His uses.

The most perfect example we have of a quiet mind in a quiet body, guided by the Divine Will, is in the character of the Lord Jesus Christ. As we study His words and His works, we realize the power and the delicacy of His human life, and we realize—as far as we are capable of realizing—the absolute clearness of the atmosphere about Him. We see and feel that atmosphere to be full of quiet—Divine Human Love.

There is no suffering, no temptation, that any man or woman ever had or ever will have that He did not meet in Himself and conquer. Therefore, if we mean to begin the work in ourselves of finding the quiet which will lay our own dust from the very first, if we have the end in our minds of truer obedience and loving trust, we can, even in the simple beginning of learning to do nothing quietly, find an essence of life which eventually we will learn always to recognize and to love, and to know that it is not ourselves, but it is from the Heavenly Father of ourselves.

Some of us cannot get that motive to begin with; some of us will, if we begin at all, work only for relief, or because we recognize that there is more power without dust than with it, but no one of us is ever safe from clouds of dust unless at the back of all our work there is the desire to give up all self-will for the sake of obeying and of trusting the Divine Will more and more perfectly as time goes on. If we are content to work thoroughly and to gain slowly, not to be pulled down by mistakes or discouragements, but to learn from them, we are sure to be grateful for the new light and warmth and power for use that will come to us, increasing day by day.

CHAPTER XXIX

Plain Every-day Common Sense

PLAIN common sense! When we come to sift everything down which will enable us to live wholesome, steady, every-day, interesting lives, plain common sense seems to be the first and the simplest need. In the working out of any problem, whether it be in science or in art or in plain everyday living, we are told to go from the circumference to the center, from the known to the unknown, from simplest facts to those which would otherwise seem complex. And whether the life we are living is quiet and commonplace, or whether it is full of change and adventure, to be of the greatest and most permanent use, a life must have as its habitual background plain every-day common sense.

When we stop and think a while, the lack of this important quality is quite glaring, and every one who has his attention called to it and recognizes that lack enough to be interested to supply it in his own life, is doing more good toward bringing plain common sense into the world at large than we can well appreciate. For instance, it is only a fact of plain common sense that we should keep rested, and yet how many of us do? How many readers of this article will smile or sneer, or be irritated when they read the above, and say, "It is all very well to talk of keeping rested. How is it possible with all I have to do? or with all the care I have? or with all I have to worry me?"

Now that is just the point—the answer to that question, "How is it possible?" So very few of us know how to do it, and if "how to keep rested though busy" were regularly taught in all schools in this country, so far from making the children self-conscious and over-careful of themselves, it would lay up in their brains ideas of plain common sense which would be stocked safely there for use when, as their lives grew more maturely busy, they would find the right habits formed, enabling them to keep busy and at the same time to keep quiet and rested. What a wonderful difference it would eventually make in the wholesomeness of the manners and customs of this entire nation. And that difference would come from giving the children now a half hour's instruction in the plain common sense of keeping well rested, and in seeing that such instruction was entirely and only practical.

It has often seemed to me that the tendency of education in the present day is more toward giving information than it is in preparing the mind to receive and use interesting and useful information of all kinds: that is, in helping the mind to attract what it needs; to absorb what it attracts, and digest what it absorbs as thoroughly as any good healthy stomach ever digested the food it needed to supply the body with strength. The root of such cultivation, it seems to me, is in teaching the practical use and application of all that is studied. To be sure, there is much more of that than there was fifty years ago, but you have only to put to the test the minds of young graduates to see how much more of such work is needed, and how much more intelligent the training of the young mind may be, even now.

Take, for instance, the subject of ethics. How many boys and girls go home and are more useful in their families, more thoughtful and considerate for all about them, for their study of ethics in school? And yet the study of ethics has no other use than this. If the mind absorbed and digested the true principles of ethics, so that the heart felt moved to use them, it might—it probably would—make a great change in the lives of the boys and girls who studied it—a change that would surprise and delight their parents and friends.

If the science of keeping rested were given in schools in the way that, in most cases, the science of ethics seems to be given now, the idea of rest would lie in an indigestible lump on the minds of the students, and instead of being absorbed, digested and carried out in their daily lives, would be evaporated little by little into the air, or vomited off the mind in various jokes about it, and other expressions that would prove the children knew nothing of what they were being taught.

But again, I am glad to repeat—if instruction, *practical* instruction, were given every day in the schools on how to form the habit of keeping rested, it would have a wonderful effect upon the whole country, not to mention where in many individual cases it would actually prevent the breaking out of hereditary disease.

Nature always tends toward health; so strongly, so habitually does nature tend toward health that it seems at times as if the working of natural laws pushed some people into health in spite of chronic antagonism they seem to have against health—one might even say in spite of the wilful refusal of health.

When one's body is kept rested, nature is constantly throwing off germs of disease, constantly working, and working most actively, to protect the body from anything that would interfere with its perfect health. When one's body is not rested, nature works just as hard, but the tired body—through its various forms of tension that impede the circulation, prevent the healthy absorption of food and oxygen, and clog the way so that impurities cannot be carried off—interferes with nature's work and thus makes it impossible for her to keep the machine well oiled. When we are tired, the very fact of being tired makes us more tired, unless we rest properly.

A great deal—it seems to me more than one-half—of the fatigue in the world comes from the need of an intelligent understanding of how to keep rested. The more that lack of intelligence is allowed to grow, the worse it is going to be for the health of the nation. We have less of that plain common sense than our grandfathers and grandmothers. They had less than their fathers and mothers. We need more than our ancestors, because life is more complicated now, than it was then. We can get more if we will, because there is more real understanding of the science of hygiene than our fathers and mothers had before us. Our need now is to use *practically* the information which a few individuals are able to give us, and especially to teach such practical use to our children.

Let us find out how we would actually go to work to keep rested, and take the information of plain common sense and use it.

To keep rested we must not overwork our body inside or outside. We must keep it in an equilibrium of action and rest.

We overwork our body inside when we eat the wrong food and when we eat too much or not enough of the right food, for then the stomach has more than its share of work to do, and as the effort to do it well robs the brain and the whole nervous system, so, of course, the rest of the body has not its rightful supply of energy and the natural result is great fatigue.

We overwork our body inside when we do not give it its due amount of fresh air. The blood needs the oxygen to supply itself and the nerves and muscles with power to do their work. When the oxygen is not supplied to the blood, the machinery of the body has to work with so much less power than really belongs to it, that there is great strain in the effort to do its work properly, and the effect is, of course, fatigue.

In either of the above cases, both with an overworked stomach and an overworked heart and lungs, the complaint is very apt to be, "Why am I so tired when I have done nothing to get tired?" The answer is, "No, you have done nothing outside with your muscles, but the heart and lungs and the stomach are delicate and exquisite instruments. You have overworked them all, and such overwork is the more fatiguing in proportion to what is done than any other form, except overwork of the brain." And the overtired stomach and heart and lungs tire the brain, of course.

Of the work that is given to the brain itself to overtire it we must speak later. So much now for that which prevents the body from keeping rested inside, in the finer working of its machinery.

It is easy to find out what and how to eat. A very little careful thought will show us that. It is only the plain common sense of eating we need. It is easy to see that we must not eat on a tired stomach, and if we have to do so, we must eat much less than we ordinarily would, and eat it more slowly. So much good advice is already given about what and how to eat, I need say nothing here, and even without that advice, which in itself is so truly valuable, most of us could have plain common sense about our own food if we would use our minds intelligently about it, and eat only what we know to be nourishing to us. That can be done without fussing. Fussing about food contracts the stomach, and prevents free digestion almost as much as eating indigestible food.

Then again, if we deny ourselves that which we want and know is bad for us, and eat only that which we know to be nourishing, it increases the delicacy of our relish. We do not lose relish by refusing to eat too much candy. We gain it. Human pigs lose their most delicate relish entirely, and they lose much—very much more—than that.

Unfortunately with most people, there is not the relish for fresh air that there is for food. Very few people want fresh air selfishly; the selfish tendency of most people is to cut it off for fear of taking cold. And yet the difference felt in health, in keeping rested, in ease of mind, is as great between no fresh air and plenty of fresh air as it is between the wrong kind of food and enough (and not too much) of the right kind of food.

Why does not the comfort of the body appeal to us as strongly through the supply of air given to the lungs as through that of food given to the stomach? The right supply of fresh air has such wonderful power to keep us rested!

Practical teaching to the children here would, among other things, give them training which would open their lungs and enable them to take in with every breath the full amount of oxygen needed toward keeping them rested. There are so many cells in the lungs of most people, made to receive oxygen, which never receive one bit of the food they are hungry for.

There is much more, of course, very much more, to say about the working of the machinery of the inside of the body and about the plain common sense needed to keep it well and rested, but I have said enough for now to start a thoughtful mind to work.

Now for keeping the body well rested from the outside. It is all so well arranged for us—the night given us to sleep in, a good long day of work and a long night of rest; so the time for rest and the time for work are equalized and it is so happily arranged that out of the twenty-four hours in the day, when we are well, we need only eight hours' sleep. So well does nature work and so truly that she can make up for us in eight hours' sleep what fuel we lose in sixteen hours of activity.

Only one-third of the time do we need to sleep, and we have the other two-thirds for work and play. This regular sleep is a strong force in our aim to keep rested. Therefore, the plain common sense of that is to find out how to go to sleep naturally, how to get all the rest out of sleep that nature would give us, and so to wake refreshed and ready for the day.

To go to sleep naturally we must learn how to drop all the tension of the day and literally *drop* to sleep like a baby. *Let go into sleep*—there is a host of meaning in that expression. When we do that, nature can revive and refresh and renew us. Renew our vitality, bring us so much more brain power for the day, all that we need for our work and our play; or almost all—for there are many little rests during the day, little openings for rest that we need to take, and that we can teach ourselves to take as a matter of course. We can sit restfully at each one of our three meals. Eat restfully and quietly, and so make each meal not only a means of getting nourishment, but of getting rest as well. There is all the difference of illness and health in taking a meal with strain and a sense of rush and pressure of work, and in taking it as if to eat that one meal were the only thing we had to do in the day. Better to eat a little nourishing food and eat it quietly and at leisure than a large meal of the same food with a sense of rush. This is a very important factor in keeping rested.

Then there are the many expected and unexpected times in the day when we can take rest and so *keep rested.* If we have to wait we can sit quietly. Whatever we are doing we can make use of the between times to rest. Each man can find his own "between times." If we make real use of them, intelligent use, they not only help us to keep rested, they help us to do our work better, if we will but watch for them and use them.

Now the body is only a servant, and in all I have written above, I have only written of the servant. How can a servant keep well and rested if the master drives him to such an extent that he is brought into a state, not where he won't go, but where he can't go, and must therefore drop? It is the intelligent master, who is a true disciple of plain common sense, who will train his servant, the body, in the way of resting, eating and breathing, in order to fit it for the maximum of work at the minimum of energy. But if you obey every external law for the health and strength of the body, and obey it implicitly, and to the letter, with all possible intelligence, you cannot keep it healthy if the mind that owns the body is pulling it and twisting it, and *twanging* on its delicate machinery with a flood of resentment and resistance; and the spirit behind the mind is eager, wretched, and unhappy, because it does not get its own way, or elated with an inflamed egoism because it is getting its own way.

All plain common sense in the way of health for the body falls dead unless followed up closely with plain common sense for the health of the mind; and then again, although when there is "a healthy mind in a healthy body," the health appears far more permanent than when a mind full of personal resistance tries to keep its body healthy, even that happy combination cannot be really permanent unless there is found back of it a healthy spirit.

But of the plain common sense of the spirit there is more to be said at another time.

With regard to the mind, let us look and see not only that it is not sensible to allow it to remain full of resistance, but is it not positively stupid?

What an important factor it should be in the education of children to teach them the plain common sense needed to keep the mind healthy—to teach them the uselessness of a mental resistance, and the wholesomeness of a clean mind.

If a child worries about his lessons, he is resisting the possibility of failing in his class; let him learn that the worry *interferes* with his getting his lesson. Teach him how to drop the worry, and he will find not only that he gets the lesson in less time, but his mind is clearer to remember it.

By following the same laws, children could be taught that a feeling of rush and hurry only impedes their progress. The rushed feeling sometimes comes from a nervous unquiet which is inherited, and should be trained out of the child.

But alas! alas! how can a mother or a father train a child to live common sensibly without useless resistance when neither the mother nor the father can do that same themselves. It is not too late for any mother or father to learn, and if each will have the humility to confess to the child that they are learning and help the child to learn with them, no child would or could take advantage of that and as the children are trained rightly, what a start they can give their own children when they grow up—and what a gain there might be from one generation to another! Will it ever come? Surely we hope so.

CHAPTER XXX

A Summing Up

GIVE up resentment, give up unhealthy resistance.

If circumstances, or persons, arouse either resentment or resistance in us, let us ignore the circumstances or persons until we have quieted ourselves. Freedom does not come from merely yielding out of resentment or unhealthy resistance, it comes also from the strong and steady focus on such yielding. *Concentration and relaxation are just as necessary one to another to give stability to the nerves of a man—as the centrifugal and centripetal forces are necessary to give stability to the Earth.*

As the habit of healthy concentration and relaxation grows within us, our perception clears so that we see what is right to do, and are given the power to do it. As our freedom from bondage to our fellowmen becomes established, our relation to our fellowmen grows happier, more penetrating and more full of life, and later we come to understand that at root it is ourselves—our own resentment and resistance—to which we have been in bondage,—circumstances or other people have had *really* nothing to do with it. When we have made that discovery, and are steadily acting upon it, we are free indeed, and with this new liberty there grows a clear sense and conviction of a wise, loving Power which, while leaving us our own free will, is always tenderly guiding us.

No one ever really believed anything without experiencing it. We may think we believe all sorts of beautiful truths, but how can any truth be really ours unless we have proved it by living? We do not fully believe it until it runs in our blood—that is—we must see a truth with our minds, love it with our hearts and live it over and over again in our lives before it is ours.

If the reader will think over this little book—he will see that every chapter has healthy yielding at the root of it. It is a constant repetition of the same principle applied to the commonplace circumstances of life, and if the reader will take this principle into his mind, and work practically to live it in his life, he will find the love for it growing in his heart, and with it a living conviction that when truly applied, it always works.

Some one once described the difference between good breeding and bad breeding as that between a man who works as a matter of course to conquer his limitations—and a man to whom his limitations are inevitable.

There is spiritual good breeding and natural good breeding. The first comes from the achievement of personal character—the second is born with us—to use or misuse as we prefer.

It is a happy thing to realize that our freedom from bondage to circumstances, and our loving, intelligent freedom from other people, is the true spiritual good breeding which gives vitality to every action of our lives, and brings us into more real and closer touch with our fellow-men. Courtesy is alive when it has genuine love of all human nature at the root of it—it is dead when it is merely a matter of good form.

In so far as I know, the habit of such freedom and good breeding cannot be steadily sustained without an absolute, conscious dependence upon the Lord God Almighty.

www.ingramcontent.com/pod-product-compliance
Lightning Source LLC
Chambersburg PA
CBHW070234190526
45169CB00001B/175